D0893604

Genetics and Life Insurance

Basic Bioethics

Glenn McGee and Arthur Caplan, editors

Genetics and Life Insurance

Medical Underwriting and Social Policy

edited by Mark A. Rothstein

The MIT Press
Cambridge, Massachusetts
London, England

This book was set in Sabon by Asco Typesetters. Printed and bound in the United States of America.

Library of Congress Cataloging-in-Publication Data

Genetics and life insurance : medical underwriting and social policy / Mark A. Rothstein, editor.
    p.   cm.
(Basic Bioethics)
Includes bibliographical references and index.
ISBN 0-262-18236-X (alk. paper)
    1. Insurance, Life—Medical examinations. 2. Genetics. 3. Bioethics.
I. Rothstein, Mark A.

HG8886.G43   2004
368.38′2012—dc22   2003064742

Printed on recycled paper.

10 9 8 7 6 5 4 3 2 1

Contents

Series Foreword

We are pleased to present the tenth book in the series Basic Bioethics. The series presents innovative works in bioethics to a broad audience and introduces seminal scholarly manuscripts, state-of-the-art reference works, and textbooks. Such broad areas as the philosophy of medicine, advancing genetics and biotechnology, end of life care, health and social policy, and the empirical study of biomedical life are engaged.

Glenn McGee
Arthur Caplan

Basic Bioethics Series Editorial Board
Tod S. Chambers
Susan Dorr Goold
Mark Kuczewski
Herman Saatkamp

Preface

It is difficult to find anyone opposed to privacy and fairness in the abstract. When one gets to the definitions of these terms and to their specific applications, then numerous divisions emerge. Imposing external notions of genetic privacy and genetic fairness on the multibillion-dollar insurance industry is a prime example. Researchers and policy analysts have found it exceedingly difficult to draft responsible recommendations that balance consumer, industry, and public interests. Fortunately, the collaborators and consultants on this book have made this seemingly arduous undertaking much easier and less contentious than one might have expected.

As anticipated, the most difficult part of the book was formulating and drafting the chapter on recommendations. A constructive and wide-ranging workshop in Chicago, with life insurance medical directors, executives, and regulators, actuaries, state legislators, lawyers, genetics experts, and consumer advocates, greatly helped to crystalize the issues. I thank all of the participants: Cathleen R. Brady, Dr. Richard Braun, Dr. Keith T. Clark, David J. Christianson, Rep. Erik R. Fleming, Dr. Robert K. Gleeson, Béatrice Godard, Dr. Joseph R. Hugenard, J. Robert Hunter, Carolyn Johnson, Rep. Phyllis Kahn, Riva F. Kinstlick, Dr. J. Alexander Lowden, Roberta B. Meyer, Dr. Michael L. Moore, Harvey Pogoriler, Sen. Sandy Praeger, Steve Radke, Dr. Bruce Rowat, Dr. Dan Scott, and Wendy Uhlmann. I also thank the following individuals for supplying information and helpful suggestions on this project: Cecil Bykerk, Cheye Calvo, Dr. Ann M. Hoven, Alissa Johnson, Joan Weiss, and Dr. Steve Zimmerman. Although I greatly appreciate their input, these individuals do not necessarily agree with all of the conclusions and recommendations in the final chapter.

Research for this book was funded by a grant from the National Human Genome Research Institute of the National Institutes of Health. I thank Dr. Jean E. McEwen of NHGRI for her support of the project. I also thank my former colleague, Elaine Lisko, for her help in drafting the original grant application.

Telesurveys Research Associates of Houston conducted the background focus groups as well as the public opinion survey. I thank Michelle Zamora for directing the focus groups. Special thanks to Rosie Zamora, Dick Jaffe, and the late Barry Petree for their help with design and administration of the survey instrument, and Dr. Eun-Sul Lee and Dr. Sharon P. Cooper for their statistical analysis.

My colleagues at the University of Louisville also played an important part in the project. Dr. Carlton A. Hornung of the School of Medicine contributed valuable data analysis and coauthored Chapter 1 of this volume. Nanette R. Elster of the Institute for Bioethics, Health Policy, and Law worked with the focus groups and helped with chapter edits. Cathy F. Rupf and Judy Oller provided flawless grant administration. Sue Rose expertly guided the manuscript through innumerable revisions.

Finally, I thank my wife, Laura, without whose support I could not have completed this or any other project.

Mark A. Rothstein
May 2003

Introduction

The year is 2020. Alan and Lisa Bennett, a couple in their twenties, are considering buying a small house and starting a family. To protect the economic security of their future child and the surviving spouse in the event of the untimely death of the other spouse, they decide to purchase life insurance. As a condition of their individual policies, Able Life Insurance Company requires them to authorize release of their medical records and to submit a blood sample. DNA extracted from the white blood cells of the sample will be tested simultaneously for the 100 most common genetic mutations associated with premature mortality. The test uses an oligonucleotide chip, similar in appearance to a computer chip. In medical practice, the chip can test for thousands of mutations and help in the prevention, diagnosis, and treatment of many illnesses. The life insurance version of the chip, which includes only life-threatening diseases, has been nicknamed "the death chip."

Alan and Lisa are not sure they want to submit a blood sample for genetic testing, because they could learn of their risks of developing disorders for which no effective treatment is available. They declined genetic testing when offered by their own physicians and, unlike some of their friends, they have not used home-collection kits to have anonymous genetic testing through mail-order laboratories advertised on the Internet. Should they be forced to submit to genetic testing to obtain life insurance? Should they have to provide a blood sample for cholesterol and other "nongenetic" medical tests? Should Able Life Insurance Company's physicians have access to family history information in their medical records from which they can infer genetic risks? Should the company be allowed to consider *any* medical information, including current health status and lifestyle, in deciding whether to issue a policy? If Alan and Lisa qualify for individual life insurance without genetic testing, should they pay the same rates as their contemporaries in poor health, or those who have had the genetic tests and have none of the risks; or should they pay some other amount?

There is one major problem with this hypothetical future. The future is here today. The chip technology is available now, although it is used mostly in research settings. The significance of a positive test for any one of the particular mutations that could be placed on a gene chip may not be clearly established, however. Consequently, few if any life insurance companies require applicants to have genetic tests. Genetic information, however, from a family history or results of a genetic test performed in the clinical setting, is now widely available in medical records and accessible to life insurers. In addition, the amount of this information in medical records will grow exponentially.

Despite the expansion of genetic knowledge and technology, from a policy standpoint, we have yet to decide the degree to which genetic information of relevance in medical settings should be available for use in other settings. We have also yet to decide whether this information should be treated the same way as other health information or whether it is somehow unique. Finally, we have yet to determine the extent to which access to results of genetic tests by third parties will dissuade people from undergoing testing.

The Human Genome Project has led to many new technologies and biological insights with great potential to improve health. It is tempting to think that new genetic discoveries raise new ethical, legal, and social implications. On closer examination, however, policy debates over genetics are dominated by concerns about such fundamental values as privacy, confidentiality, and fairness. As in other areas in which society is debating the proper role of genetics, sound policy for genetics and life insurance is proving to be inseparable from sound policy for life insurance in general.

This book draws on the talents and perspectives of a wide range of contributors to explore the proper policies for genetics and medical underwriting in life insurance. It includes results of the nation's first comprehensive survey of public opinion on genetics and life insurance, as well as contributions from a representative of the trade association for life insurance companies, an actuary, an insurance physician, a geneticist, a philosopher, a genetic counselor together with the president of a genetics consumer organization, a dean and professor of insurance law, a trio of comparative law researchers, and an insurance consumer advocate. The book concludes with a series of policy recommendations designed for adoption long before 2020.

Contributors

Mark A. Rothstein, J.D., Editor
Herbert F. Boehl Chair of Law and
Medicine
Director, Institute for Bioethics,
Health Policy and Law
University of Louisville School of
Medicine

Norman Daniels, Ph.D.
Professor of Ethics and Population
Health
Harvard School of Public Health

Arnold A. Dicke, FSA, MAAA, EA
Principal
Bell & Dicke LLC

Robert K. Gleeson, M.D., FACP
Vice President and Medical Director
Northwest Mutual Life Insurance
Company

Béatrice Godard, Ph.D.
Projet Genetique et Societe, Centre de
Recherche en Droit Public
University of Montreal

Carlton A. Hornung, Ph.D., M.P.H.
Professor and Acting Chair, Depart-
ment of Epidemology & Clinical
Investigational Sciences
University of Louisville School of
Public Health and Information
Sciences

J. Robert Hunter
Director of Insurance
Consumer Federation of America

Robert H. Jerry II, J.D.
Dean and Levin, Mabie & Levin
Professor of Law
Frederic G. Levin College of Law
University of Florida

Yann Joly, LL.B.
Projet Genetique et Societe, Centre de
Recherche en Droit Public
University of Montreal

Bartha Maria Knoppers, LL.D.
Projet Genetique et Societe, Centre de
Recherche en Droit Public
University of Montreal

J. Alexander Lowden, M.D., Ph.D.
Lab One Canada

Roberta B. Meyer, J.D.
Senior Counsel
American Council of Life Insurers

Sharon F. Terry, M.A.
President, Genetic Alliance
Executive Director, PXE International

Wendy R. Uhlmann, M.S., C.G.C.
Genetic Counselor/Clinic Coordinator
University of Michigan

Genetics and Life Insurance

1

Public Attitudes

Mark A. Rothstein and Carlton A. Hornung

When the Human Genome Project officially began in 1990, the first social concern to generate widespread interest was the possibility that health insurance companies would use predictive genetic information to charge individuals higher rates or to exclude them from coverage (Murray 1992; NIH-DOE Working Group 1993). Both the public sentiment of strong opposition to such practices and the public policy response of enacting legislation prohibiting genetic discrimination in health insurance were easy to predict. Although comprehensive federal bills to prohibit genetic discrimination in health insurance have languished in Congress, the Health Insurance Portability and Accountability Act of 1996 (HIPAA) prohibits employer-sponsored group health plans from excluding from coverage, charging higher rates, or offering different benefits to members of a group based on their genotype (HIPAA 1996). In addition, all but a few states have enacted laws prohibiting genetic discrimination in health insurance, applicable mostly to individual policies and nonemployer groups (Hall 1999; National Conference of State Legislatures 2001).

As the policy focus has shifted to the possible role of genetic information in life insurance underwriting, it is important to consider public attitudes about a range of related questions. What does the public regard as the primary social function of life insurance? What is the proper role of underwriting in general? If individuals learn that they are at a genetically increased risk of developing a serious illness in the future, would this affect their decision to purchase life insurance or the amount of coverage? If individuals are concerned about genetic discrimination in life insurance, how does the level of concern compare with other social concerns? What, if any, legislative action would be appropriate to deal with the issue?

This chapter reports some of the key findings of the first comprehensive public survey on genetic information and life insurance underwriting. In general, the data lead to the following four conclusions: (1) the public generally believes that life insurance companies would use genetic information to deny coverage or charge higher rates; (2) individuals who learned that they were at a genetically increased risk of a serious illness would be more likely to buy all forms of insurance, but especially health and disability insurance; (3) the likelihood of purchasing all forms of insurance on learning of a genetically increased risk is strongly correlated with age, with younger individuals most likely to be purchasers; and (4) support for legislative limitations on the use of genetic information by life insurers is most correlated with education level, with people with the most education supporting such measures.

Prior Research

As with the policy analysis and legislative activity, public opinion research on genetics and insurance has concentrated on health insurance. Four data sources on public attitudes regarding genetics and life insurance, however, are worth exploring: a 2002 Harris poll, two empirical research studies on adverse selection in life insurance (Zick et al. 2000; Armstrong et al. 2003) and data from an interview survey generated by our research team in 2001.

An interactive telephone survey of 1,013 adults was conducted between May 15 and 21, 2002 (Harris 2002). Among the questions asked was the following:

If you were given a genetic test which showed how likely you were to get one or more serious diseases, which of the following do you think should be allowed to see this information?

The results, originally published in the *Wall Street Journal*, were as follows:

Your regular doctor	90%
Any doctor who is helping you to prevent a disease for which the test shows you are at risk	69%
Your health insurance company which is paying the cost of this treatment or care	39%

A life insurance company from which you want to obtain
life insurance   25%
Your employer who is paying for part of your health
insurance   17%
Not sure/refused   5%

The question has two interesting elements. First, it asked who
should be able to see the information. Although it did not ask whether
insurance companies, for example, should be able to use results of the
genetic tests in deciding coverage or rates, a likely interpretation by
many respondents was that having access to the information could lead
to some (possibly adverse) action. Second, life insurance companies are
the only entities on the list that are not involved in providing or reim-
bursing for health services. Even with these caveats, the 25% figure is
consistent with our earlier surveys reported below.

The second major piece of research attempted to measure the actions
of at-risk individuals rather than general public opinion. Zick et al.
studied 105 women age eighteen to fifty-five years from a large kindred
who had undergone research genetic testing to determine whether they
were carriers of a breast cancer mutation (BRCA 1). Of these women,
twenty-eight tested positive and seventy-seven tested negative. A control
group consisted of 177 women from the general population who had not
had genetic testing but who had at least one first- or second-degree relative with breast or ovarian cancer. The study followed the women for
one year to ascertain whether they differed in life insurance-purchasing
behavior based on genetic information. In other words, would a
woman's knowledge of her genetically increased risk of breast cancer
lead her to purchase more life insurance or adverse selection?

The authors found no differences in the number of life insurance policies purchased or coverage levels between women in the study kindred
and those from the general population. Neither family history, testing
status, nor participation in prior BRCA 1 research studies had an effect
on purchasing life insurance. The authors recognized, however, that the
study had some clear limitations, including at least the following: (1) the
Utah study population was quite homogeneous and consisted largely of
active members of the Church of Jesus Christ of Latter Day Saints; (2)
only twenty-eight women tested positive; and (3) the one-year follow-up
period may have been too short. Nevertheless, at a minimum, the study

failed to find evidence that adverse selection in life insurance would be an immediate and widespread reaction to knowledge of a genetically increased risk of breast cancer in an at-risk family.

Third, another study assessed the effect of genetic testing for breast cancer risk on the life insurance purchasing behavior of women in a university-based breast cancer clinic from 1995 to 2000 (Armstrong et al. 2003). Surveys were mailed to 1,186 women, 926 who had participated in the clinical risk assessment program and 262 who had tested positive for a BRCA1/2 mutation through a research testing protocol. The questionnaires asked about current life insurance coverage, changes in life insurance made since going through the program, and occurrence of life insurance discrimination since participation in the risk assessment. A total of 709 questionnaires were returned, but only 636 respondents were deemed eligible for inclusion in the final study cohort.

Almost half the women expressed concern about future life insurance discrimination if they underwent genetic testing, and this fear was a leading reason for refusal to undergo testing. Despite the fear, however, there was no evidence of actual discrimination. Thirty-seven women (6%) reported changing their life insurance coverage after genetic testing or counseling, with twenty-seven increasing coverage, six decreasing or canceling coverage, and four not specifying their action. Women who increased their coverage were more likely to have tested positive for a BRCA1/2 mutation.

The study authors noted the following limitations of their research. Patients were drawn primarily from a single clinical site in Philadelphia, the sample size was small, and the survey relied on self-reports of life insurance purchasing behavior. In addition, there was no control group of women who did not enter the breast cancer risk evaluation program.

Finally, as part of research on pharmacogenomics (Rothstein 2003), we conducted a nationwide telephone interview survey of 1,796 individuals in 2001. We asked the following questions (on a rotating basis):

If your employer could get the results of a genetic test that showed whether you were more likely to get sick in the future, what impact, if any, would this have on your willingness to take the test?

If your health insurance company could get the results of a genetic test that showed whether you were more likely to get sick in the future, what impact, if any, would this have on your willingness to take the test?

If your life insurance company could get the results of a genetic test that showed whether you were more likely to get sick in the future, what impact, if any, would this have on your willingness to take the test?

Approximately 70% of respondents said that disclosing test results to a third party would make them less likely to take a genetic test. Unlike the Harris survey, responses in our survey were quite similar for employers, health insurers, and life insurers. Using multivariate analysis, we determined that being white, having a higher income, and having more education correlated with a lower likelihood of undergoing testing if results were available to employers, health insurers, or life insurers (Rothstein and Hornung 2003).

Methodology

The current survey consisted of randomly dialed telephone interviews with 2,108 individuals across the country between January 3 and April 14, 2002. The research was funded by a grant from the National Human Genome Research Institute of the National Institutes of Health. Interviews were conducted by Telesurveys Research Associates of Houston, Texas, under contract with the Institute for Bioethics, Health Policy, and Law of the University of Louisville School of Medicine.

Before conducting the interviews, sessions were held with four focus groups composed of white, African-American, Hispanic, and Asian individuals. The focus groups explored levels of awareness, knowledge, and opinions concerning genetic testing and use of genetic information in life insurance underwriting. They also provided an opportunity to assess individuals' comprehension of concepts and issues and to document the vocabulary used to describe these concepts and issues.

With the aid of focus group findings, the survey instrument was drafted by the principal investigator and survey contractor. After several revisions, the instrument was pretested in twenty interviews for length (under 15 minutes) and clarity. The final instrument was translated and back-translated by separate translators into Spanish, Mandarin and Cantonese Chinese, Vietnamese, and Korean. The research protocol and survey instrument received approval from the Human Studies Committee of the University of Louisville. All interviewees gave oral consent at the beginning of the interview.

A two-stage sampling design was created with an overall sample of 2,108, with oversampling to achieve a minimum subgroup size of 300 for whites, African-Americans, Hispanics, and Asians. The first stage consisted of a primary sample of 1,500 interviews completed by random digit dialing to all area codes in the forty-eight contiguous states, with the number interviewed in direct proportion to population. A total of 608 additional interviews were conducted to increase the sample size to a minimum of 300 for each of the four racial-ethnic groups. This was accomplished by targeted random digit dialing from area codes and telephone exchanges in which 30% or more of households were of the designated racial-ethnic group. Race and ethnicity designations were based on self-identification; respondents also could designate "other," but only a small number chose to do so. Therefore this category is not reported in findings in which race and ethnicity are reported.

This sampling design yielded both widespread geographic representation and inclusion of households with listed and unlisted telephone numbers. Furthermore, the sample of 2,108 yielded estimates with a margin of error of only 2.14% at the 95% confidence level, and 90% statistical power for detecting racial-ethnic pairwise differences of 6% at alpha equals 0.05.

The investigators recognize that Hispanics and Asians are heterogeneous groups. The preferred sampling methodology would have used oversampling to include a sufficient number of Chinese-Americans, Vietnamese-Americans, Japanese-Americans, Korean-Americans, Filipino-Americans, and other Asian subpopulations to detect important differences. Similarly, the preferred methodology would have used oversampling for Mexican-Americans, Cuban-Americans, Puerto Rican-Americans, and other Hispanic subpopulations. Native Americans also would have been included and sampled in sufficient numbers. Financial constraints, however, necessitated limiting the survey to four racial and ethnicity categories.

Telephone interviews were conducted in English, Spanish, Chinese, Vietnamese, and Korean. Up to five contact attempts were made for each telephone number at different times of day. The response rate for residential calls where the call was answered (not counting businesses, fax machines, or voice mail) was 68.3%.

The survey contained sixteen substantive questions, most with sub-parts, that asked respondents about their current life insurance coverage, their perceptions of how insurers and individuals would be likely to respond to predictive genetic information, and their opinions on public policy options to address the issue. The survey used the following fifteen demographic variables: household size, age, education, marital status, employment status, residence in urban or rural area, race-ethnicity, language spoken at home, country of birth, religion, income, prior genetic testing, health status, and gender (appendix 1.1).

Key Findings

The survey findings present a wealth of information. In this chapter, we report on the following five areas of inquiry: (1) public opinions about the expected action of life insurance companies if they have access to genetic information; (2) likely insurance-purchasing behavior of individuals who learn they are at a genetically increased risk of a serious health problem; (3) public opinions on possible regulation of use of genetic information by life insurance companies; (4) public concerns about genetic discrimination relative to other issues; and (5) public views about the need for life insurance. All data analyses were accomplished using Statistical Package for the Social Sciences (SPSS) software. Cases were weighted by age for all racial-ethnic comparisons and by race-ethnicity for all age comparisons. All other analyses used a case-weighting system to reflect both age and race-ethnicity, with sample weights adjusted to yield a total of 2,108 cases.

Expected Action of Life Insurance Companies if They Have Access to Genetic Information

Although little documented evidence of adverse treatment of individuals in employment (Miller 2000), health insurance (Hall 1999) or life insurance (Zick et al. 2000) exists to date, concern about discrimination is widespread. Such concern should not be dismissed as irrational and unworthy of consideration for two important reasons. First, the amount of predictive genetic information in medical records is expected to grow tremendously as medical applications of genetic research move beyond rare, monogenic disorders to more common, multifactorial, chronic diseases. Second, the fear of discrimination already is causing many at-risk individuals to forgo genetic testing, thereby failing to take advantage of the opportunity for prevention and early diagnosis. Thus, there is an important population health component of concern about discrimination.

We attempted to measure public attitudes regarding the likely effects of genetic information on policy issuance and pricing by life insurance companies. We asked: "Now I would like to find out what you think life insurance companies might do if they have access to genetic information. If a life insurance company has access to the genetic information of someone applying for a life insurance policy, do you think they would be likely to. . . ." Subjects were asked to respond yes, no, or don't know to each of the following options: refuse to sell the policy; agree to sell the policy at the regular price; agree to sell the policy at a higher price; and agree to sell the policy at a lower price; refusals also were noted.

Because life insurance is a highly competitive business and companies attempt to sell as many policies as possible (Meyer 2004), in theory, the effect of additional genetic (or other predictive medical) information would be neutral on overall availability and pricing of life insurance. Thus, for example, one could argue that for every individual whose rates were raised from standard rates on the basis of being considered at a high risk, another individual's rates would be lowered due to assumed low risk. Even if this assumption is correct, upward and downward adjustments in price are unlikely to be made on an equal-number basis. For example, a few individuals might be offered insurance at much higher rates (or not at all), and many individuals would have the same or only slightly lower rates.

In general, the public believes that genetic information would result in life insurance companies refusing to issue policies (85.1%) or charging higher premiums (85.1%). Only 26.7% said that companies would agree to sell the policy at the regular price, and only 19.5% said that genetic information would result in the issuance of a policy at a lower price.

As shown in figure 1.1, significant differences were found across racial-ethnic groups in beliefs about what life insurance companies would do if they had access to genetic information. More than 90% of whites said that they thought companies would refuse to sell a policy and that they

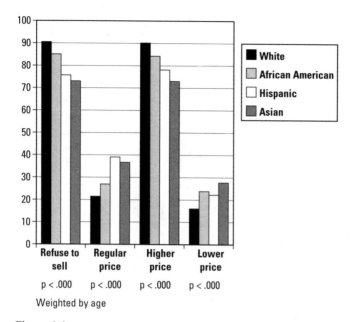

Figure 1.1
Perception of life insurers' likely response to genetic information, by race/
ethnicity.

would charge a higher price, whereas only about 72% of Asians held
these views. At the same time, whites were least likely to think that companies would sell a policy at the regular or lower price, whereas Asians
and Hispanics were most likely to say that would be the case.

Important differences were revealed in beliefs depending on the age of
the respondent (figure 1.2). The youngest and oldest respondents were
least likely to believe that insurance companies would refuse to sell a policy or charge a higher price, but more than 90% of those between ages
35 and 64 years believed this would occur. At the same time, between
80% and 90% of respondents in each age group thought that insurance
companies would sell policies at higher prices.

As shown in figure 1.3, the percentage of respondents who thought
insurance companies would deny a policy or sell it at a higher price if
they had access to genetic information increased with income. In contrast, the percentage thinking that insurance policies would be sold at the
regular price decreased with income. Finally, respondents earning
between $25,000 and $74,999 per year were least likely to believe that

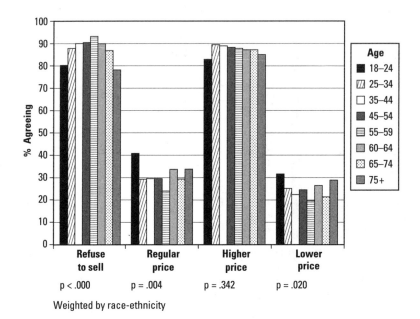

Figure 1.2
Perception of life insurers' likely response to genetic information, by age.

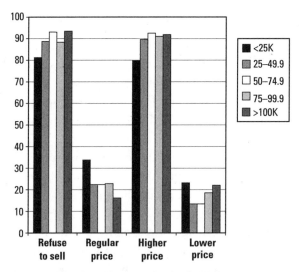

Figure 1.3
Perception of life insurers' likely response to genetic information, by income.

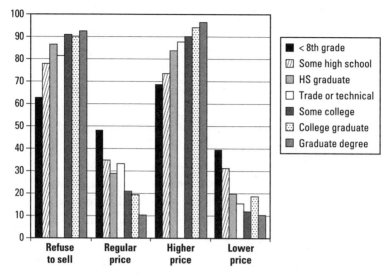

All < .000; weighted by age and race-ethnicity

Figure 1.4
Perception of life insurers' likely response to genetic information, by education.

companies would sell policies at a reduced price if they had genetic information about applicants.

Education had the clearest relationship to what respondents believed about how life insurance companies would act if they had access to an individual's genetic information (figure 1.4). The percentage who believed that insurance companies would refuse to sell a policy and the percentage who thought companies would sell a policy at a higher price increased with years of education. Between 60% and 70% of those with less than an elementary education, but over 90% of those with a graduate degree, thought this way. As expected, the percentage who thought that an insurance company would sell a policy at the regular price or at a lower price decreased with education from a high of about 40% among those with an elementary education or less to less than 10% with a graduate degree.

Beliefs about Genetic Information about Disease and Consumers' Insurance Purchasing Behavior
The greatest threat to risk-based insurance of any type is adverse selection, defined as the likelihood that those who know they are at increased

risk will be more likely to purchase insurance and in greater amounts than those who lack such knowledge or know they are at decreased risk (Dicke 2004; Gleeson 2004; Pokorski 1995). Insurers attempt to prevent adverse selection in various ways, including the obvious example of refusing to sell flood insurance to homeowners after a hurricane has been tracked bearing down on the coast.

Adverse selection has two essential elements in the context of medical underwriting. First is asymmetry of information relevant to mortality risks. If the insurance company has the same predictive health information as the consumer, known risks can be reflected in the pricing of the product. Currently, few genetic tests are performed in routine medical practice, and they are generally limited to testing for predisposition to rare disorders among individuals with a family history of the illnesses. Because life insurance application forms ask about family health history, as to rare disorders there is unlikely to be substantial information asymmetry between the applicant and the company. The possibility of asymmetry will grow, however, as more genetic tests are performed for more common disorders in primary care settings or even by applicants themselves if home-collection genetic test kits become more widely available.

The second requirement for adverse selection is the inclination of an individual to act on the information, willingness to "game the system" by withholding information in the medical underwriting process. Virtually no empirical evidence or survey data of likely consumer behavior are available in the specific context of genetic information and life insurance. One empirical study found no evidence of adverse selection (Zick et al. 2000) and another study found some evidence of adverse selection (Armstrong et al. 2003), but both studies had serious methodological limitations.

We asked respondents if they thought that consumers would withhold unfavorable results of a genetic test from a life insurance company. Nearly one-fourth (23.1%) strongly agreed and 50% agreed, whereas only 11.3% disagreed or strongly disagreed. Almost three-quarters of the population believe that other people would withhold information from an insurance company about a genetic test that indicated that they were more likely to get a serious illness. When half of the sample was asked if they agreed or disagreed with the statement that "it would be wrong to withhold genetic information from an insurance company," just 50.6% agreed or strongly agreed, 25.9% disagreed, and 5.8% strongly disagreed. The other half of the sample was asked if they agreed or disagreed that it "would *not* be wrong to withhold genetic information from a life insurance company"; 37.7% disagreed or strongly disagreed, but 43.3% agreed and 10.9% strongly agreed.

To summarize these findings, respondents overwhelmingly expected consumers to withhold unfavorable results of a genetic test from life insurers. They were more closely divided on the issue of whether it would be wrong to do so, with results varying on whether the question was asked in the affirmative or negative.

We attempted to obtain additional insights into the prospects of adverse selection in life insurance based on genetic information by asking a question that placed life insurance in the context of other forms of insurance. We asked the following:

I am going to read a list of different types of insurance and ask you to tell me whether you would be likely or unlikely to buy each type if a medical test indicated you were at an increased risk of getting a serious disease. First, if a medical test indicated that you, personally, had an increased chance of getting cancer or heart disease in the next ten years, would you be likely or unlikely to (buy/buy more) ...

A. Health insurance?
B. Life insurance?
C. Long-term care or nursing home insurance?
D. Disability insurance that would pay a portion of your wages if you could not work due to accident or illness?

Before stating the responses, a few words of explanation. We believed it was necessary to give an example of some common, serious illnesses so that all respondents would use a similar definition of "serious illness." We chose cancer and heart disease, the former because it is an area where several genetic tests already are in use and the latter because it is the most common cause of mortality. We included the ten-year figure so that all respondents would be applying the same time horizon. Based on results of focus groups, we thought it necessary to add brief explanations of long-term care and disability insurance, but did not think it necessary to explain health or life insurance. The order in which insurance products were mentioned was rotated. Finally, the answer options for each question were likely, unlikely, and unsure; refusals also were noted.

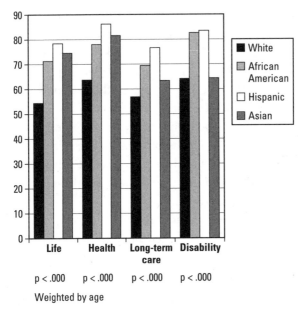

Figure 1.5
Likelihood of buying life insurance if medical test indicated increased 10-year risk of cancer or heart disease, by race/ethnicity.

Overall, respondents indicated an interest in purchasing all forms of insurance, with the following specific percentages: health 70.6%; disability 70.3%; long-term care 62.8%; and life 61.1%. Although the question did not ask whether respondents would also refuse to divulge to the insurance company that they had undergone testing, the answers shed light on this point. Figure 1.5 presents responses according to race-ethnicity. Hispanics were most likely to respond that they would buy or buy more insurance if they had information about an increased risk of illness (88.6% health, 85.5% disability, 80.5% life, 78.8% long-term care) and whites were least likely to do so (health 65.5%, life 56%, long-term care 58.3%, disability 65.8%). The high percentage of Hispanic respondents may be explained by the fact that they were the group least likely to have life insurance in the first place, only 45.0%, compared with 77.9% for African-Americans, 75.6% for whites, and 47.5% for Asians.

Perhaps surprising, in light of the role of predictive information affecting insurance-purchasing behavior, figure 1.6 indicates that the likeli-

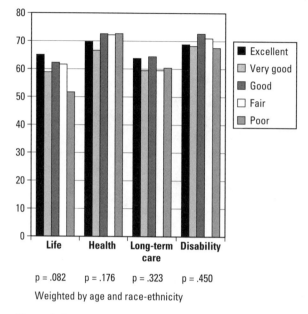

Figure 1.6
Likelihood of buying life insurance if medical test indicated increased 10-year risk of cancer or heart disease, by health status.

hood of an individual buying insurance is not affected by current health status. Similarly, neither education nor income was a significant predictor of likelihood to buy or buy more insurance. Figure 1.7, however, indicates a strong association between age and likelihood of buying life, health, and disability insurance, with younger individuals much more likely to buy or buy more insurance. On the one hand, this may not be viewed as great a risk of adverse selection because younger individuals are less likely to have insurance at the outset, and the amount they would purchase is likely to be lower because they generally have lower incomes and fewer assets. On the other hand, the result may be viewed as a substantial risk of adverse selection because younger people pay much lower premiums for life insurance because of their lower mortality risk, and premature death in this cohort would result in a substantial loss in expected years of life. The percentage saying they would be likely to buy any type of insurance did not differ according to either education or income.

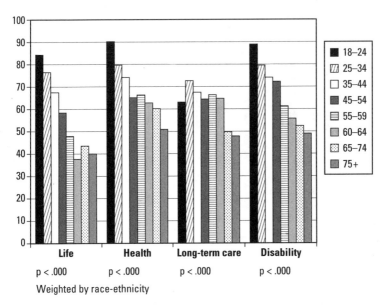

Figure 1.7
Likelihood of buying life insurance if medical test indicated increased 10-year risk of cancer or heart disease, by age.

Opinions on Possible Regulation of Life Insurers' Use of Genetic Information

Elected officials, executives of the life insurance industry, academics, consumer advocates, and numerous other individuals have begun searching for an appropriate response to the issue of genetic information and life insurance underwriting. We attempted to identify public opinion about various policy options. The immediate options available to life insurance companies are to acquire relevant genetic information from an applicant's medical record, or to require someone applying for a policy to take a specific genetic test or a battery of tests to determine risk of life-threatening disease. To explore beliefs about what the population thinks is appropriate genetic information that an insurance company should be allowed to obtain, we asked:

Now I am going to read some general statements about life insurance and genetic testing and ask whether you agree, disagree, or have no opinion. The first is . . .

A. Life insurance companies should be allowed to require all applicants to take a genetic test.

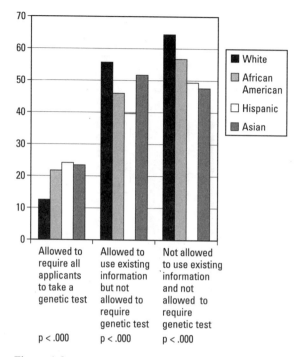

Figure 1.8
Preference for regulation of life insurers' use of genetic information, by race/
ethnicity.

B. Life insurance companies should not be allowed to use either the results of
genetic tests or other genetic information.
C. Life insurance companies should be able to use genetic information from
existing medical records, but they should not be allowed to require applicants to
take a genetic test.

The order in which the three parts of the question were asked was
rotated. The answer options were agree, no opinion, disagree, and
unsure; refusals also were noted.

Most respondents (60.8%) said that life insurance companies should
not be permitted to use *either* the results of genetic tests or other genetic
information. Most (53.2%) said that companies should be able to use
genetic information from existing medical records, but they should not
be allowed to require applicants to take a genetic test. Only 15.4%
agreed with the statement that companies should be allowed to require
all applicants to take a genetic test. As shown in figure 1.8, whites

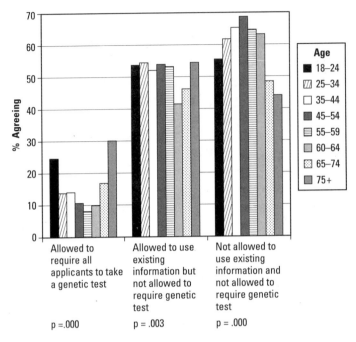

Figure 1.9
Preference for regulation of life insurers' use of genetic information, by age.

(12.4%) were least likely to say that companies should be allowed to require applicants to take a genetic test and most likely (55.6%) to say that companies should be allowed to use existing information.

Figure 1.9 reveals the effect of age on the answers. Between 25% and 30% of respondents less than twenty-four and over seventy-five years of age were most likely to approve of required genetic testing. Socioeconomic status characteristics also appear to be important determinants of attitudes. More than 20% of the lowest-income group said that insurance companies ought to be allowed to require applicants to have a genetic test, but only about 8% of the highest-income group had that opinion (figure 1.10). Similarly, between 25% and 30% of respondents who did not complete high school approved of life insurance companies requiring genetic tests, compared with less than 10% of respondents who had a college or graduate degree (figure 1.11). When it came to using existing genetic information from an applicant's medical record, clear differences of opinion were seen by education, but less clear differences

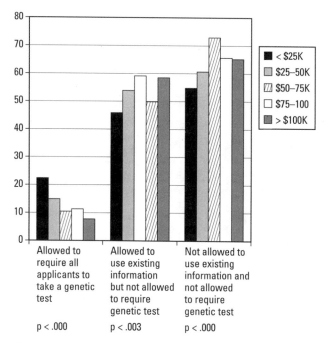

Figure 1.10
Preference for regulation of life insurers' use of genetic information, by income.

by economic status. Respondents with the least education were least likely to say that companies ought to be allowed to use existing information. In contrast, groups with the highest education were twice as likely to allow companies access to existing information.

What is interesting to note is that the lowest-education group, those with less than an elementary education and who presumably had the least understanding of genetic testing and genetic information and what they can be used for, did not seem to distinguish between the implications of requiring a test and using existing information. However, as education level increased, respondents were more likely to oppose required genetic tests but would permit use of genetic information that might already exist.

Figure 1.12 provides counterintuitive results. We asked individuals if they ever had a genetic test, and those who had *not* had a genetic test were most likely to oppose allowing life insurance companies to require such tests. Although it is not clear what is responsible for this result, it

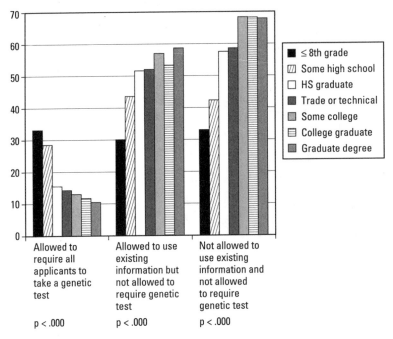

Figure 1.11
Preference for regulation of life insurers' use of genetic information, by education.

may be that it reflects negative test results or individuals who had declined testing because of possible nonmedical uses of the information. It also should be noted that only 8.1% of respondents reported having had a genetic test.

Concerns about Genetic Discrimination Relative to Other Issues

In our earlier interview survey on public attitudes toward pharmacoge-nomics we learned that the public is concerned about the possibility of genetic discrimination (Rothstein and Hornung 2003). Although this finding is consistent with numerous studies, it does not measure the degree of concern about genetic discrimination relative to other matters. We tried to address this issue in the current study. As the first part of a question, we asked the following:

Are you concerned that, as scientists learn more about genetics, there is likely to be genetic discrimination or making decisions against a person based on his or her genetic information rather than their actual health?

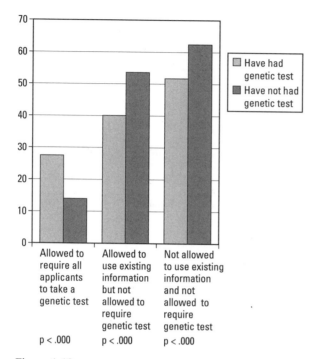

Figure 1.12
Preference for regulation of life insurers' use of genetic information, by whether they have had a genetic test.

Not surprising, 83.1% of respondents answered yes. In part two of the question, we asked those who answered yes the following:

I am going to read a list of other issues and ask you to tell me whether you feel each one is a bigger concern or a smaller concern than genetic discrimination. If you feel any of the issues and genetic discrimination are equal concerns, please tell me that. First,...

We gave them a list of seven concerns that we asked in rotating order: cloning, crime, the economy, the environment, access to health care, taxes, and terrorism (figure 1.13). About five times more respondents rated terrorism, crime, access to health care, and the economy as causing more concern than rated genetic discrimination a concern. The environment was a more important concern than genetic discrimination by a margin of about three to one, and taxes by a margin of two point five to one. Even cloning, which had the lowest level of concern of the comparison issues, was more a concern than genetic discrimination by a margin of four to three.

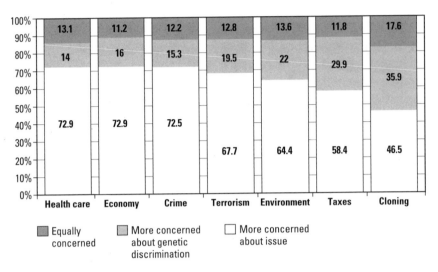

Figure 1.13
Concern about genetic discrimination relative to other issues.

Thus, genetic discrimination, although reported as a concern by 83.1% of respondents, was less a concern than any of the other items on the list. It should be noted that we asked about genetic discrimination in general, which could include employment, health insurance, and other forms of discrimination.

The Need for Life Insurance

A major policy question for possible regulation of the use of genetic information in life insurance (and a recurring theme in several of the chapters that follow) is whether access to life insurance should be considered an economic issue or a civil rights issue. If the former, insurance companies should be given wide latitude in deciding what information to consider in underwriting. If the latter, restricting insurer prerogatives (with the effect of low-risk individuals subsidizing high-risk individuals) may be necessary to promote other social policies. As described below, the survey data also may shed some light on public views on this question.

We asked the following:

Now I am going to read some statements about insurance and ask you to tell me whether you strongly agree, agree, have no opinion, disagree, or strongly disagree with each one. The first statement is …

A. Everyone needs health insurance.
B. Everyone has a right to health insurance.
C. Everyone needs life insurance.
D. Everyone has a right to life insurance.

The questions were block rotated (A and B, C and D). Because there is no legal right either to health or life insurance, we assumed that questions B and D were viewed by respondents as "Everyone should have a right to health/life insurance."

Of our respondents, 91.2% said that everyone needs health insurance and 90.6% said that everyone has a right to it. These data were in line with expectations. Furthermore, 69.2% said that everyone needs life insurance. This was in line with expectations (70% of households have life insurance), in that depending on age, health, family status, and financial status, a substantial minority of respondents might not believe that everyone needs life insurance. On the second part of the question, however, instead of a comparable response, as was the case with the question on health insurance, 82.6% of respondents said that everyone has a right to life insurance. Overall, 62.2% agreed with both statements—that everyone needs and should have a right to life insurance.

A wide range of demographic factors can be detected from these responses. Those who regarded life insurance as both a need and a right had fewer years of education, tended to be African-American or Hispanic, were Catholic, and had total family incomes under $25,000 per year. About 20% believed that everyone needs life insurance, but that it is not a right. These individuals were likely to have college or postgraduate education, be older and widowed, be white or Asian, and have an annual income over $100,000. A little less than 7% did not feel that everyone needs life insurance, but that they should have a right to it. They were likely to be retired and to have incomes above $75,000 per year. Finally, about 10% of respondents did not think that everyone needs life insurance and did not believe that everyone should have the right to it. These individuals completed the most education, were more likely to be white, and to have incomes above $50,000.

How does one account for this disparity? Consistent responses regarding health insurance were not repeated for life insurance. A substantial number of respondents had different opinions about whether access to life insurance is an economic issue (need insurance), a civil rights issue (have a right to insurance), both, or neither. The remaining chapters address both aspects of life insurance, and the recommendations in chapter 11 focus on these concerns.

Conclusion

The interview survey provides a detailed look at public attitudes about the use of genetic information in life insurance underwriting. The following conclusions can be drawn from the data: (1) most people expect life insurers to use genetic information to deny coverage or increase rates; (2) those who learn that they are at an increased risk of having a serious illness are most concerned about obtaining health and disability insurance; (3) age is the most significant factor affecting the likelihood of purchasing insurance after learning about an increased health risk; (4) most individuals are opposed to life insurers requiring applicants to take a genetic test as a condition of obtaining a policy; and (5) whereas overwhelming concern was expressed about genetic discrimination, it is considerably behind all other social issues we probed.

References

Armstrong, K., "Life Insurance and Breast Cancer Risk Assessment: Adverse Selection, Genetic Testing Decisions, and Discrimination," Am. J. Med. Genet. 120A: 359–364 (2003).

Dicke, A. A., "The Economics of Risk Selection in Life Insurance," in Genetics and Life Insurance: Medical Underwriting and Social Policy, M. A. Rothstein, ed. Cambridge: MIT Press (2004).

Gleeson, R., "Medical Underwriting for Life Insurance," in Genetics and Life Insurance: Medical Underwriting and Social Policy, M. A. Rothstein, ed. Cambridge: MIT Press (2004).

Hall, M., "Legal Rules and Industry Norms: The Impact of Laws Restricting Health Insurers' Use of Genetic Information," Jurimetrics J., 40: 93–125 (1999).

Harris Interactive, "Americans Say They'd Use Genetic Testing for Diseases," Wall St. J., June 5, 2002.

Health Insurance Portability and Accountability Act, 42 U.S.C. §§300gg-300gg-2 (1996).

Meyer, R., "Genetics and Life Insurance: The Insurer Perspective," in Genetics and Life Insurance: Medical Underwriting and Social Policy, M. A. Rothstein, ed. Cambridge: MIT Press (2004).

Miller, P., "Is there a Pink Slip in My Genes? Genetic Discrimination in the Workplace," J. Health Care Law & Policy 3: 225–245 (2000).

Murray, T., "Genetics and the Moral Mission of Health Insurance," Hastings Center Rep., 22(6): 12–17 (1992).

National Conference of State Legislatures, Denver and Washington, D.C.: National Conference of State Legislatures, Genetics Policy Report: Insurance Issues (2001).

NIH-DOE Working Group on Ethical, Legal, and Social Implications of Human Genome Research, Genetic Information and Health Insurance, Report of the Task Force on Genetic Information and Insurance (1993).

Pokorski, R., "Genetic Information and Life Insurance," Nature 376: 13–16 (1995).

Rothstein, M. A. ed., Pharmacogenomics: Social, Ethical, and Clinical Dimensions. Hoboken, N.J.: John Wiley & Sons (2003).

Rothstein, M. A. and C. A. Hornung, "Public Attitudes About Pharmacogenomics," in Pharmacogenomics: Social, Ethical, and Clinical Dimensions," M. A. Rothstein ed. Hoboken, N.J.: John Wiley & Sons (2003).

Zick, C. et al., "Genetic Testing, Adverse Selection, and the Demand for Life Insurance," Am. J. Med. Genet. 93: 29–50 (2000).

2

The Insurer Perspective

Roberta B. Meyer

Risk classification based on medical underwriting lies at the core of the existing voluntary, private life insurance business. In large part it is this process that enables insurers to make life insurance products widely available at affordable prices in the United States.

The Life Insurance Market

Life insurance is a financial product. People buy it to protect their future financial security and to protect their dependents against financial hardship when they die. Many life insurance products also allow policy holders to accumulate savings that can be used in time of financial need. Sixty-nine percent of families owned some type of life insurance in 1998, the most recent year for which this statistic is available (American Council of Life Insurers [ACLI] 2001, p. 93).

The need for private life insurance protection continues to grow. Americans purchased $2.7 trillion worth of new coverage in 2000, 7% more than in 1999. By the end of 2000, total life insurance coverage in the United States reached $16 trillion, up $457 billion, or 3% over 1999 (ACLI 2001, pp. 93–94).

Three types of life insurance policies predominate. Individual insurance is sold and underwritten on an individual basis. Group insurance is underwritten on a group of people as a whole, such as employees of a company or members of an organization. Credit insurance guarantees payment of some form of credit, such as a mortgage or other loan, in the event the insured person dies. It can be bought on either an individual or group basis.

Individual life insurance is the most widely purchased form of protection. It is typically purchased through agents and issued through policies with face amounts of at least $1,000, although larger minimum amounts are common in today's market. Individual policies are principally used for family protection, but also for business purposes. A business may purchase life insurance to protect against economic loss that would result from the death of the owner or key employee. At the end of 2000, individual life insurance accounted for 59% of all life insurance in force in the United States (ACLI 2001, pp. 94–95).

Individual life insurance protection in the United States rose to $9.4 trillion at the end of 2000, up 2% from $9.2 trillion in 1999. It has grown at an average annual rate of 6% since 1990, when $5.4 trillion was in force. The size of newly purchased policies also continued to rise in 2000, on average growing 12% to $134,800, compared with $119,000 in 1999 and $75,300 in 1990 (ACLI 2001, pp. 95–96).

Individual policies provide two basic types of protection. Term policies insure an individual for a specified period of time or term. Permanent or whole life policies insure an individual for his or her entire life.

In 2000, 87.4% of applications for individual life insurance policies resulted in policies that were issued and paid for, 8.3% of these applications resulted in offers for coverage that were declined by the applicant, and only 4.3% were declined by insurers (ACLI 2001, p. 108). In the same year, over 21% of policies were issued at preferred-risk rates, accounting for 52% of the face amount of coverage issued. Seventy-five percent of policies were issued at standard rates, accounting for 43% of the face amount issued; and 5% were issued at substandard (or extra-risk) rates (ACLI 2001, pp. 107, 109).

Risk classification enables insurers to take advantage of a number of factors that contribute to the high rate of acceptance of applicants. Improvements in medicine, job safety, and public health make possible issuance of coverage at standard and preferred rates previously not possible. Similarly, sale of extra-risk policies, issued to individuals in poor health or hazardous occupations at higher than standard premiums, make it possible for some people to obtain coverage they could not have purchased in the past.

The Risk Classification Process

The process of risk classification serves insurers, policy holders, and applicants for coverage (or proposed insureds) by perpetuating financial soundness and fairness. As explained in detail in another chapter, through risk classification and underwriting, insurance companies place applicants into groups or classes. Each class consists of individuals who pose the same or comparable levels of risk. All members of a class pay the same premium. In this way, insurers assure that premiums are appropriate to risks and that all those with the same level of risk pay the same premiums.

In 1980, the American Academy of Actuaries Committee on Risk Classification developed a statement of principles according to which the three primary purposes of a risk classification system are "to protect the insurance program's financial soundness; be fair; and permit economic incentives to operate and thus encourage widespread availability of coverage" (p. 2). Elimination or severe restriction of risk classification would thwart these goals, thereby jeopardizing the existing private life insurance system.

Protection of Financial Soundness

Risk classification assures that premiums are financially prudent or adequate to enable the insurer to meet its contractual obligations to its policy holders. It allows the insurer to determine premiums that are appropriate to levels of risk. The more underwriting information available to the insurer, the more precise it can be in determining appropriate premiums. This protects both insurer and policy holders from the insurer becoming insolvent due to inadequate premiums.

Adverse Selection

A fundamental purpose of insurance underwriting and risk selection is to protect both insurers and policy holders from adverse selection (or antiselection). An individual who knows he or she is going to be sick or die prematurely may have a strong incentive to purchase new or larger amounts of insurance than he or she would have otherwise. The individual also has a strong incentive to withhold unfavorable health information from the insurer to which he or she is applying. Unfortunately, not all applicants are honest about their medical history or status. In the absence of complete medical information, the insurer is likely to put such an individual in an inappropriately low premium class. Initially, this will result in unfair subsidization of that individual by other insureds. Ultimately, if enough insureds withhold negative information, it could jeopardize the financial viability of the insurer.

If the insurer is unable to assess risks fully and accurately, it could have a number of results. The price of coverage for healthy people would be likely to increase, perhaps uncontrollably, to compensate for claims of unhealthy people. Many people with a legitimate need for insurance, who would qualify for coverage under customary standards, might refrain from purchasing insurance because of the increased cost, needlessly depriving their families of coverage. Finally, a dramatic withdrawal of healthy persons from a particular insurer or from the market altogether could lead to the collapse of that insurer or the insurance system.

Some observers refuse to believe that adverse selection is real unless they see evidence of it. Examples arise due to misrepresentations in relation to tobacco and drug use and HIV infection status, where the number and amount of claims were dramatically higher than they would have been in the absence of antiselection. However, it is difficult or impossible to find evidence of severely damaging adverse selection in connection with life insurance in the last 100 years. This is true because insurers have not thus far been deprived of the means with which to control it.

Whereas a few cases of adverse selection might not have a significant negative impact on the market, many cases industry-wide would. This would be particularly true if individuals were legally permitted to withhold or restrict access to genetic information or results of genetic tests that exist at the time of application, that have a significant bearing on the likelihood of premature death, and that might influence the timing, nature, and amount of coverage sought. Laws to this effect would legalize practices that currently constitute fraud and material misrepresentation (and protect insurers and consumers against adverse selection). Ultimately, the major negative consequence of adverse selection would be to drive up costs for future customers that could price many average American families out of the life insurance market.

Fairness

Risk classification ensures that all of an insurer's applicants and existing policy holders are treated fairly. This is required by the National Association of Insurance Commissioners (NAIC) model Unfair Trade Practices Act (UTPA) and by the unfair discrimination statutes, based on the UTPA, in effect in all fifty states. These statutes are strongly supported by the industry.

Section 4 of the UTPA reads in pertinent part as follows:

> Any of the following practices ... are hereby defined as unfair trade practices in the business of insurance:
>
> ...
>
> G. Unfair Discrimination.
> (1) Making or permitting any unfair discrimination between individuals of the same class and equal expectation of life in the rates charged for any life insurance policy or annuity or in the dividends or other benefits payable thereon, or in any other of the terms and conditions of such policy (NAIC).

To avoid unfair discrimination and to treat all applicants and all existing policy holders fairly, insurance companies must set premiums at a level consistent with the risk represented by each proposed insured. For them to be able to do this, relevant and available cost-effective information must be considered. Insurance, by its very nature, requires distinction among individuals. Underwriting is properly performed and discrimination is fair when the proposed insured's expected future mortality and morbidity have been properly estimated and reflected in decisions regarding whether to issue coverage and, if so, the premium rate.

Unfair discrimination, on the other hand, is not and should not be permitted. In insurance underwriting it occurs when equal risks are treated differently. In other words, it occurs when no sound actuarial justification or reasonably anticipated claims experience can justify the manner in which risks are classified, or when an underwriter misclassifies a risk because a relevant piece of information is kept from consideration.

Legislators in all fifty states have acknowledged their understanding and appreciation of the necessity for fair discrimination in insurance underwriting by enacting statutes with language similar, if not identical, to that of section 4 the UTPA. Like the UTPA, these statutes require that insurers treat persons of the same class in the same way, prohibiting unfair and implicitly requiring fair discrimination. The existence of these statutes eliminates the need for legislation to govern or to ensure fairness on the basis of genetic tests or genetic information.

The industry would support an explicit requirement that underwriting on the basis of genetic information or tests results must be fair, meaning that it must be "based on sound actuarial principles or ... related to actual or reasonably anticipated experience" (NAIC Model Regulation 1979). In fact, the industry would support a requirement that *all* medical underwriting be subject to this standard. Several states have amended unfair trade practices acts to incorporate this or similar language.

This language is derived from the NAIC Model Regulation on Unfair Discrimination in Life and Health Insurance on the Basis of Physical or Mental Impairment which reads in pertinent part as follows:

> The following are hereby identified as acts or practices in life and health insurance which constitute unfair discrimination between individuals of the same class: refusing to insure, or refusing to continue to insure, or limiting the amount, extent or kind of coverage available to an individual, or charging a different rate for the same coverage solely because of a physical or mental impairment, except where the refusal, limitation or rate differential is based on sound actuarial principles or is related to actual or reasonably anticipated experience.

Operation of Economic Incentives

Life insurers have incentives to seek potential customers and to sell and service those customers to expand their markets and to achieve high penetration in the markets. This works to the advantage of consumers as well, because it allows premiums to remain affordable, making coverage widely available.

Some seeking to limit insurers' use of genetic information maintain that such legislation is necessary to prevent creation of a genetic underclass. They conclude that without such restrictions, insurers will use genetic test results or genetic information to refuse coverage to as many people as they can. This concern is ill founded, as evidenced by the fact that genetic discrimination feared in connection with health insurance never materialized.

Moreover, insurers have no desire to turn away business. They attempt to offer coverage to as many people as possible while assuring themselves that their prices are adequate to fulfill future contractual obligations to policy holders. Also, it is largely because prices are affordable that these products are widely available.

The process of risk classification protects insurers and existing policy holders by ensuring that premiums are financially prudent and by providing a shield against adverse selection. It also protects applicants by ensuring fairness in underwriting. It allows insurers to operate in a free, competitive market, resulting in affordable prices and, consequently, in widely available coverage. This voluntary, private system could not continue to exist in the absence of such a framework.

Importance of Risk Classification

Risk classification is critically important to all individually underwritten life insurance products. It is no less important to policies with face amounts of $5,000 than it is to those with face amounts of $5 million. In connection with all policies, regardless of size, the same need exists "to protect the insurance program's financial soundness; be fair; and permit economic incentives to operate ..." (American Academy of Actuaries 1980). This need is met under the current system through risk classification. Some advocates suggest prohibiting use of broadly defined genetic information in underwriting for policies up to a specified minimum amount of coverage. If enacted into law, these proposals would require a fundamental restructuring of a major part of the current market in the United States. These proposals are strongly opposed by the industry.

A law based on such a proposal would skew much of the current market, making it highly vulnerable to adverse selection, since individuals would have no incentive to purchase life insurance until they were sick. By permitting applicants to withhold adverse medical information material to the likelihood of premature death, it would legalize practices that constitute fraud or material misrepresentation under current law, further undermining protections against adverse selection. It would grant a constructive entitlement to a specified minimum amount of life insurance and guarantee coverage for certain individuals, giving them preferred status over people with unprotected medical conditions.

One proposal suggested prohibiting use of genetic information in connection with underwriting for policies with face amounts up to

$100,000, with the implication that that is a basic amount of life insurance coverage. In fact, the average face amount is $134,800 (ACLI 2001, pp. 95–96). So, again, this proposal would undermine medical underwriting for much of the existing individual life insurance market in this country.

Also, some insurers sell only policies with relatively small face amounts. Medical underwriting by these insurers would be significantly (if not totally) undermined by such a proposal. In addition, schemes that would permit consumers to purchase several policies totaling a certain maximum amount of coverage with limited or no underwriting generally fail to provide who or what entity would be charged with monitoring when someone has reached the permissible limit.

Use of Genetic Information in Risk Classification for Life Insurance

Distinguishing between Genetic Information and Other Medical Information and Genetic Tests and Other Medical Tests

We have no generally accepted definitions of the terms "genetic information" or "genetic tests." It is widely recognized that it is not easy to distinguish between genetic and nongenetic diseases. Indeed, as we learn more about the genetic mechanisms of disease, we are finding it increasingly difficult to make such distinctions.

In the spring of 1993, the Task Force on Genetic Information and Insurance of the NIH-DOE Working Group on Ethical, Legal, and Social Implications of Human Genome Research delivered a report on genetic information and health insurance. This report stated: "As a practical matter, it will become increasingly difficult to deal with genetic information as special and separate from other forms of health related information because diseases are increasingly understood as having both genetic and environmental components" (Task Force 1993, p. 3). Furthermore:

Recognizing that our genes affect many common diseases not previously thought of as genetic will transform the scope and meaning of terms such as genetic information, genetic test, asymptomatic condition, presymptomatic condition, and genetic predisposition to disease.

Important and common diseases are coming to be understood as a complex mixture of genetic and non-genetic factors.

It is important to recognize the difficulty (if not impossibility) of distinguishing genetic information and tests from other medical information and tests. It is also important to recognize that, because they serve different purposes, legislative definitions of these terms may differ from scientific definitions. Moreover, certain definitions may be appropriate for use only in connection with underwriting limits or requirements in relation to certain types of insurance products. For example, definitions developed in connection with underwriting limits for health insurance (taking into account practices specific to health insurers) are probably inappropriate in connection with rules or requirements applicable to underwriting for life insurance.

In sum, the life insurance industry strongly questions both the necessity for legislation limiting the use of genetic information or genetic test results in connection with life insurance, and the feasibility of crafting underlying legislative definitions of genetic information and genetic tests that appropriately distinguish genetic information and tests from other medical information and tests. However, if such legislation is unavoidable, life insurers urge that the terms "genetic information" and "genetic test" be carefully defined to *include* information pertaining to and tests of only the individual seeking coverage and not family members, and to *exclude* traditional medical information and tests, including routine medical tests and physical measurements; tests commonly accepted in clinical practice; diagnostic or prognostic tests; tests measuring manifestations of existing disease; and information as to the results of these tests and measurements.

Use of Genetic Information in Underwriting for Life Insurance

Insurers have used broadly defined genetic information in underwriting for a long time. Applications for policies commonly seek information on family history, cholesterol level, hypertension, coronary heart disease, cancer, diabetes, and many other impairments that may have a genetic basis, which is inherited, acquired, or both. Many applicants are requested to undergo blood and other tests for conditions or diseases such as high cholesterol that may have a genetic component. Insurers' right to evaluate and to underwrite on the basis of information from these tests is essential to risk classification.

Insurers' Approach to DNA-Based Technologies

The report of the NIH-DOE task force commented on the impending genetic revolution, stating a "[a] wave of new genetic information is coming ..." (Task Force 1993, p. 4). Others are making this same prediction. Although such a wave has not yet been sighted, insurers sense its presence and are concerned. Life insurers believe that this technology must be dealt with in an intelligent and rational manner.

The industry has not rushed to embrace narrowly defined, DNA-based genetic tests. In fact, insurers are approaching them very cautiously in their usual approach to technological advances. As stated, they generally refrain from requiring medical tests in underwriting until the tests have been shown to be reliable. Although no insurers are known to require genetic tests as part of the underwriting process, questions have arisen because of rapidly developing scientific advances, various legislative challenges, and inquiries such as that being conducted by the study underlying this book.

When applicants undergo such tests in clinical settings before applying for insurance coverage, it is critical that insurers have access to and the right to underwrite on the basis of test results in order to avoid adverse selection. If the number of DNA-based tests administered in clinical settings increases as anticipated, this will become increasingly important, as the results of these tests are likely to influence the timing, nature, and amount of coverage sought.

Privacy Issues

The industry is well aware that consumers have privacy concerns in relation to confidentiality and security of personal information and heightened concerns about medical information, including genetic information. Insurers believe that all personal medical information should be given the same high level of confidentiality and security protection. They believe that each consumer wants such information to be confidential and secure, regardless of whether it is characterized as genetic information. Life insurers strongly support the NAIC Insurance Information and Privacy Protection Model Act, the NAIC Model Privacy of Consumer Financial and Health Information Regulation, and the NAIC Standards for Safeguarding Customer Information Model Regulation.

By its very nature, life insurance involves personal and confidential relationships, and it is imperative for insurers to maintain consumers' trust in these relationships. The ACLI's adoption and strong support of the following principles of support for use in connection with legislative and regulatory proposals, reflects industry's appreciation of this imperative:

1. Medical information to be collected from third parties for underwriting life, disability income and long-term care insurance coverages should be collected only with the authorization of the individual.

2. In general, any redisclosure of medical information to third parties should only be made with the authorization of the individual.

3. Any redisclosure of medical information made without the individual's authorization should only be made in limited circumstances, such as when required by law.

4. Medical information will not be shared for marketing purposes.

5. Under no circumstances will an insurance company share an individual's medical information with a financial company, such as a bank, in determining eligibility for a loan or other credit—even if the insurance company and the financial company are commonly owned.

6. Upon request, individuals should be entitled to learn of any redisclosures of medical information pertaining to them which may have been made to third parties.

7. All permissible redisclosures should contain only such medical information as was authorized by the individual to be disclosed or which was otherwise permitted or required by law to be disclosed. Similarly, the recipient of the medical information should generally be prohibited from making further redisclosures without the authorization of the individual.

8. Upon request, individuals should be entitled to have access and correction rights regarding medical information collected about them from third parties in connection with any application they make for life, disability income or long-term care insurance coverage.

9. Individuals should be entitled to receive, upon request, a notice which describes the insurer's medical information confidentiality practices.

10. Insurance companies providing life, disability income and long-term care coverages should document their medical information confidentiality policies and adopt internal operating procedures to restrict access to medical information to only those who are aware of these internal policies and who have a legitimate business reason to have access to such information.

11. If an insurer improperly discloses medical information about an individual, it could be subject to a civil action for actual damages in a court of law.

12. State legislation seeking to implement these principles should be uniform. Any federal legislation to implement the foregoing principles should preempt all other state requirements.

It is noteworthy that whereas insurers strongly support these principles, they must still be permitted to obtain, use, and share customers' personal health information to perform legitimate business functions. These functions are essential to life insurers' ability to serve and meet their contractual obligations to their existing and prospective customers.

Applications for life insurance seek nonmedical information, such as age, occupation, income, net worth, and social security number. They also ask questions that focus on the proposed insured's health, including routine measurements, such as height and weight, blood pressure, and cholesterol level; current medical conditions and past illnesses; injuries; and medical treatments. The insurer may also request evaluation of blood, urine, or other specimens, including tests for tobacco or drug use or HIV status.

Often the applicant is asked to provide the name of each physician or practitioner consulted in connection with any ailment within a specific period or time (typically five years). It should be reiterated that no life insurers are known to require genetic tests, and none is known explicitly to request information about the results of such tests performed outside the context of insurance before application for coverage. However, if an individual has undergone a genetic test, it is expected that that information will be provided. Depending on the person's age and medical history, and the amount of coverage applied for, information from medical records or additional financial data (assets, estate-planning goals) may be required.

Once an insurer has an applicant's personal health information, it limits access to that information. Different insurers use different mechanisms to protect both confidentiality and security of consumer information and to meet requirements of extensive federal and state privacy laws and regulations. Within this framework, insurers must use and sometimes share personal medical information to perform legitimate business functions— to underwrite the applications of prospective customers, to pay claims, to administer and service existing contracts, and to perform related product or service functions.

In sum, the industry is strongly committed to the principle that individuals have a legitimate interest in the proper collection and handling of their personal information, including medical information, and that insurers have an obligation to assure individuals of the confidentiality and security of that information. Life insurers believe that all consumer medical information should be afforded the same high level of confidentiality and security protection.

Myths and Fears in Relation to Life Insurance and Genetics

Myths

Several myths relate in one way or another to discussions about genetic information and life insurance. The first deals with the linkage between the terms "genetics" and "heredity." When people hear the phrases genetic disease or genetic test, most automatically think of inherited disease or tests for them. Whereas this would have been correct a few years back, scientists are learning that most if not all diseases have a molecular basis and that genetic disorders may be either inherited or acquired. Both genetically inherited and acquired conditions are likely to be significant to medical underwriting for a life insurance policy depending on their nature and the proposed insured's other medical characteristics.

Take cancer as an example. All cancers are genetic. They originate from a single cell that becomes malignant because the cellular DNA is transformed by a carcinogen or environmental factor. In addition, the tendency to develop some cancers is inherited. For example, 5% of breast cancers are caused by known, inherited genetic mutations; the other 95% are also genetic, but are overwhelmingly acquired somatic mutations.

Another disease that is not considered to be genetic is AIDS, although it is in a certain sense. When the AIDS virus enters human cells it inserts itself into the DNA or genome of those cells. This transforms or mutates the cells' DNA and converts the cells into virus producers. Thus genetic changes induced by a virus are the cause of HIV disease.

The second myth deals with the widely held misperception that genetic tests are always concerned with future rather than present disease. DNA-based genetic tests designed to diagnose cancers and other diseases by definition deal with conditions that are already present. They aid in early diagnosis of disease that already exists.

Genetic tests are being developed to define the genetic makeup of a tumor or disease-causing organism and to design therapies tailored to those genetic characteristics. For example, genetic tests are performed on the microorganism that causes tuberculosis to determine if a given *Mycobacterium* is resistant to conventional drug therapy.

Another prognostic genetic test involves polymerase chain reaction testing of blood to detect malignant cells that are in the process of metastasizing from a primary site to distant body locations. The results may signal an unexpected need for aggressive chemotherapy. Because results of both diagnostic and prognostic genetic tests provide information relevant to the likelihood of premature death, they are likely to be critical to medical underwriting.

A third myth underlies much of the debate over insurers' use of genetic information and relates to the proposition that it is unfair for insurers to underwrite on the basis of conditions over which individuals have no control. Such a proposition reflects lack of understanding of risk classification. The function of risk classification is not to make value judgments with respect to certain behaviors but to evaluate levels of risk. Many, if not most, diseases are beyond an individual's control. Moreover, there is no single view regarding the meaning of factors that *are* within an individual's control. Finally, given the blurring of the distinction between genetic and other medical conditions, the issue of whether a disease or condition is within an applicant's control is likely to become moot.

A fourth myth derives from the view that it is unfair for insurers to underwrite on the basis of genetic tests that indicate that healthy persons will develop disease in the future. This proposition too reflects a fundamental misunderstanding of risk classification. The process evaluates the possibility or probability, not the certainty, of a proposed insured contracting disease or dying prematurely. Life insurance underwriters use diagnostic tests, prognostic tests, and tests that measure predisposition to disease to assess the likelihood of the applicant's premature death. In fact, they are concerned only with existing disease to the extent that it does (or does not) indicate a risk of premature death.

The proposition that it is unfair to underwrite on the basis of healthy individuals' possibility of future disease also reflects lack of understanding of the important distinction between being presymptomatic versus being predisposed to a disease. However, the fact that an individual is either presymptomatic of or predisposed to a disease is likely to have actuarial significance.

The term "presymptomatic" signifies early disease, not wellness. When insurers began testing for the HIV antibody in 1985–1986, it was often argued that an asymptomatic person who tested positive looked and felt well and should be treated as such. Insurers made the counter-argument that AIDS typically was associated with an initial multiyear asymptomatic period, followed by a second stage called AIDS-related complex, then by full-blown AIDS, followed by death. The most appropriate term for this sequential process was "HIV disease." The fact that a proposed insured with HIV disease was presymptomatic was not material to an actuarial assessment of the risk posed by that applicant or his or her likelihood of premature death.

This same concept applies to Huntington disease, which is a late-onset inherited disease. A thirty-year-old who is tested and confirmed to carry the Huntington disease mutation may not develop symptomatic neurodegenerative disease for another ten to twenty years. Average persons this age are expected to live another fifty years, but this thirty-year-old will probably die in half that time. This difference in expected life span clearly is material to actuarial assessment.

Many inherited diseases are caused by a complex interaction of multiple genes and environmental factors. Coronary artery disease is a good example. If individuals inherit alleles that predispose them to high cholesterol and hypertension, they are predisposed to prematurely developing serious coronary disease, although they may or may not become ill. Similarly, persons who have perfectly normal cholesterol levels and blood pressure (and presumably normal genes for these factors) are predisposed to good health, but can develop coronary disease.

Analysis of an applicant's predisposition to disease relates to probabilistic considerations as to whether the person will contract disease or die prematurely. Insurers treat conditions such as high blood pressure and elevated cholesterol as though they were shades of gray. They do not assume that someone with hypertension will have a heart attack, but they know that the probability of heart disease is increased. The individual's level of risk or possibility of premature death is probabilistically judged to be increased and therefore must be considered in underwriting.

Thus, to be complete and fair, underwriters must be able to take into account relevant information in relation to a proposed insured's medical history and current disease as well as information indicating that the individual may be presymptomatic of or have a predisposition to a disease. All of this information has actuarial significance indicating likelihood of premature death.

A fifth myth pertains to what might be termed the one-sided coin. When people hear the term genetic testing, they often think of abnormal results and unfavorable consequences. Such a focus is unfortunate. The fact is that most tests, and genetic tests will be no exception, yield a vast preponderance of normal results and a small minority of abnormal results. If it proves to be true, as many now are predicting, that genetic screening for conditions such as breast cancer and myriad other conditions will eventually become standards of medical practice, millions of Americans will receive reports from their doctors that they are not at increased risk for a number of diseases. It is possible that these test results could make otherwise uninsurable individuals insurable, or make it possible for many of them to obtain coverage at cheaper rates.

Fears

Some fear that if they test positive for a genetic condition they will never be able to obtain life insurance, and that if one insurer declines their application for coverage, others will do the same. In fact, this is not necessarily the case. To the contrary, a positive test result certainly does *not* necessarily mean that an individual will not be able to obtain life insurance coverage. As noted earlier in this chapter, currently, the vast majority of individuals who apply for life insurance are issued coverage at standard or better rates and there is no evidence to indicate that this is going to change.

The fact is that underwriters take a proposed insured's complete medical history and status into account, not just the results of a single test. Moreover, over 1,500 life insurers are doing business in the United States. Different ones use different criteria when determining who to insure and at what price. If an individual is turned down by one company, he or she probably will be able to obtain coverage from another. Also, it is possible that if a company declines an application as a result of a condition that goes away or improves, the person may be able to obtain coverage even with that insurer at a later time.

Some fear that life insurers are anxious to start using DNA-based genetic tests and to require them as a prerequisite of coverage. The truth is that life insurers are rarely, if ever, on the forefront of science in their adoption of new technologies. They use only tests that meet certain reliability and specificity standards. They recognize that, for the most part, DNA-based genetic tests are new and unproved. Based on available information, life insurers do not order applicants to undergo DNA-based genetic tests.

Concern exists that as genetic technology improves, the constant increase in the number of genetic tests and number of genes identified as contributing to disease will cause many Americans to become uninsurable. In the long run, it is likely that advances in genetic science, like technological advances of the past, will make life insurance coverage available to those who could not obtain it before, and enable others to purchase coverage more cheaply than they could have otherwise. This is the case for those with cardiovascular disease and diabetes, early diagnosis and treatments of which allow people to live longer, making them candidates for insurance when they were not before.

Some people are concerned that if a genetic test indicates that they have a particular disorder that insurers will cancel existing policies or increase the rates. That is not possible. As long as premiums continue to be paid, life insurers are contractually bound to maintain coverage and may not increase premiums, due to any deterioration in the insured's health or the outcome of any medical tests, including DNA-based genetic tests, performed after coverage has gone into effect. It is noteworthy that in some cases, premiums may be decreased if the insured's health improves.

Conclusion: Industry Perspectives on Policy

Depending on its nature and breadth, a prohibition or limitation of underwriting for life insurance on the basis of genetic information or the results of genetic tests could jeopardize risk classification and consequently, the vibrancy and health of the market. For this reason, the issue is fundamentally important to insurers and to the millions of American families that depend on life insurance to assure their future financial security. The industry does not believe that legislation limiting its use of genetic information or tests in connection with life insurance is necessary.

Insurers recognize that revolutionary advances in genetic technology and their heralding in the press have given rise to public fears in relation to the use of such information. They know of the fear that genetic information or tests will be used to cancel or deny insurance coverage or to increase rates. In the past, most of this fear related to concern regarding the availability and affordability of health insurance. In fact, over the past decade, fear of genetic discrimination in connection with health insurance drove much of the public discourse (and most legislative initiatives) in relation to genetics and insurance. It is significant that it is now generally acknowledged that this did not occur. And insurers contend that such fears in connection with life insurance are without foundation.

Risk classification and selection is only successful when all risks are placed in the correct groups. Technology and medical advances have helped drive the price of insurance down in two ways: by improving mortality, and by helping insurers to assess risk more accurately. There is no reason to think that advances in genetics should not continue that trend. (Zimmerman 1998)

Life insurance is a financial product generally sold and underwritten on an individual basis. While health insurance is purchased to provide indemnity for costs of medical care, life insurance is purchased to protect families' future financial security.

Individual life insurance policies are likely to be in effect for decades. Once a policy is issued, it may not be canceled, nor may the premium be increased due to deterioration in the insured's health or the results of medical tests performed after issuance of coverage. Because insurers get essentially "one bite at the apple" during the underwriting process to assess the risk of premature death accurately, it is critical that medical information be as complete and accurate as possible.

Life insurers' most fundamental concern in relation to genetic information is that it not result in a proposed policy initiative that would intentionally (or inadvertently) jeopardize traditional medical underwriting on the basis of traditional medical information or traditional medical tests. Growing knowledge of the complexity of interrelationships between the genetic and environmental components of disease make it unclear whether it is possible to distinguish between genetic information and other medical information and genetic tests and other medical tests. Proposed definitions often intentionally or unintentionally include traditional information and tests that have been used in and are critical to underwriting. If enacted into law, limits on underwriting based on such broadly defined terms could undermine traditional medical underwriting and require fundamental structural changes in the market.

It is critical that no legislation jeopardize or impair insurers' ability to access and underwrite on the basis of relevant medical information existing at time of application, and likely to influence the timing, nature, and amount of coverage sought. This is true regardless of whether existing information is traditional or genetic, or derived from a traditional or genetic test. It is necessary to protect insurers and their millions of existing and potential customers from possible significant effects of adverse selection.

If a limitation on life insurers' right to require genetic tests were unavoidable, the industry would strongly urge that it not be permanent (so that insurers' practices would not be legislatively frozen in time forever preventing them from giving their customers the benefit of future advances); genetic tests be defined to exclude routine medical tests and physical measurements, tests commonly accepted in clinical practice, diagnostic or prognostic tests, and those measuring manifestations of existing disease; and it not be required that a genetic test be on a list of approved tests before it may be used, which would be unworkable at the present time for a variety of reasons discussed below.

Life insurers believe it is inappropriate to single out a particular type of information for a high level of privacy protection. The ACLI principles of support relating to confidentiality of medical information make no distinction between individuals' genetic and other medical information. Among other things, the principles include support for legislative/regulatory proposals providing for insurers' collection of medical information from third parties only with authorization of the individual, limits on disclosure of medical information by insurers, and prohibitions on insurers' sharing medical information for marketing purposes or for determination by a financial company of eligibility for a loan or other credit.

In considering public policy and developing possible legislative proposals in relation to life insurers' use of genetic information or the results of genetic tests, it is critical to determine the ultimate goal(s) and to ascertain ramifications of new initiatives. For example, legislation that would limit or prohibit underwriting on the basis of genetic information, defined broadly enough to include traditional medical information, would have profound implications for risk classification and require a fundamental restructuring of the current market. The same is true regarding a proposal intended to guarantee a certain minimum amount of private life insurance at standard rates for all individuals, regardless of their medical or genetic status or history. By contrast, a proposal to limit insurers' ability to require narrowly defined DNA-based genetic tests, while still objectionable to insurers, would have a more circumscribed effect.

The vibrancy of the life insurance marketplace, reflected by widespread availability and affordability of insurance in the United States, is made possible and perpetuated by risk classification regulated by and permitted under the regulatory framework. It is not evident that we need or that consumers desire its restructuring. Nor is there evidence of a need for more narrow limits on underwriting, such as a moratorium or prohibition on insurers' right to require genetic tests.

Historically, advances in science and technology have made it possible for people to live longer and for insurers better to assess the likelihood of premature death. Advances in genetic science are predicted to have the same salutary effect.

References

American Academy of Actuaries Committee on Risk Classification, "Risk Classification Statement of Principles," (1980).

American Council of Life Insurers, ACLI 2001 Life Insurers Fact Book (2001).

Task Force on Genetic Information and Insurance, NIH-DOE Working Group on Ethical, Legal, and Social Implications of Human Genome Research, "Genetic Information and Health Insurance," (1993).

NAIC Model Unfair Trade Practices Act, initially adopted in 1947, as amended in 2001.

National Association of Insurance Commissioners, Model Regulation on Unfair Discrimination in Life and Health Insurance on the Basis of Physical or Mental Impairment; Section 3 (1979).

Zimmerman, S. E., "The Use of Genetic Tests by Life Insurance Companies: Does this Differ from the Use of Routine Medical Information," Genetic Testing 2: 3–6 (1998).

3

The Economics of Risk Selection

Arnold A. Dicke

Risk selection has always been an integral part of insurance. Insurance by its nature is a contract, and to settle the terms of a contract, information is necessary. Even in ancient days when goods were sent over the seas in wooden boats, it was impossible to find a party to provide indemnity cover for the shipment without providing that party with information regarding the value of the items, destination, route, and other matters that affected risk. Some risks were thought to be too severe for anyone to provide insurance; others carried a price that seemed to someone to be appropriate compensation.

Processes by which prices emerge are the subject of microeconomics. Contract formation and the role of information are among subjects studied by a newer branch of economics, information economics, or game theory. Insurance is an important source of examples for microeconomic theorists and information economists alike, since trade-offs inherent in insurance transactions touch aspects of human behavior not usually so clearly on display. The practical implications of these economic analyses of insurance are the province of actuarial science.

Although for many insurance transactions both potential insurer and potential insured have the same information (or uncertainty about information), in other situations the potential insured has the advantage of greater knowledge of conditions that could affect the insured risk than the insurer has, unless detailed investigations are undertaken. This disparity in knowledge about risk is an example of what economists call information asymmetry. Information asymmetry exists whenever one party to a transaction has greater or different information than the other party. A particular type of information asymmetry that often affects insurance transactions is adverse selection: one party has information before the transaction that would change the terms of the transaction if known to the other party. Insurance contracts are also affected by another form of information asymmetry—moral hazard, which occurs when an insured person changes his or her behavior after an insurance contract is made.

Most economic analysis of insurance focuses on coverages, such as many property-casualty and health coverages, that indemnify specific losses and usually involve a contract that is in effect renegotiated annually. Both characteristics simplify analysis of contract formation.

Life insurance and the life insurance market have economic characteristics that distinguish them from property-casualty coverages and their markets. In life insurance, some aspects of the risks undertaken may appear more predictable than most property-casualty and health risks. After all, all persons will die some day, whereas a fire or a shipwreck might be avoided indefinitely; and the benefit to be paid under life insurance is fixed in advance. However, life insurance is a timing risk, and the actual cost of the benefit on a present value basis emerges only with the passage of years or even decades. The contract is designed to stay in force until the benefit would be paid and usually provides for premiums to be paid over an extended period, perhaps for the remaining life of the insured. Also, underlying reasons for a person's obtaining life insurance coverage are more diverse, and thus the amounts necessary to indemnify the risks are harder to determine than for other types of insurance. These and other differences identified below mean that adverse selection plays an even more significant role in life insurance than in short-term coverages, and the social benefit from the optimizing dynamic of the marketplace is even greater.

Finally, life insurance involves information and events that are more personal than those associated with property and casualty coverages. Because of this, intervention through subsidies or other mechanisms may be requested to minimize the impact that the freely operating life insurance market may have on individuals. Also, concern about the dependence of the value of inforce life insurance contracts on the insureds' longevity prospects has largely prevented emergence of a secondary market for such contracts.

These considerations mean that, whereas the same tools of economic analysis can be applied to life insurance as to other coverages, appropriate adaptations must be made. Care must be taken and explicit and implicit assumptions checked before the results of such analysis are carried over to life insurance.

Assessment Societies—Inability to Reflect Known Risks in a Noncancelable Arrangement

Economic analysis can provide a formal structure for discussion and examination of the fundamental problem caused by differences in life expectancy found in any group of potential insured lives. This problem emerged most dramatically in the failure of nineteenth-century institutions called assessment societies. These groups were based on the correct perception that because an individual's time of death is uncertain (even more so in that era of infectious diseases and limited medical and surgical remedies), risk could be moderated through pooling of resources. To pay a predetermined benefit on the death of any member of the society to the deceased's beneficiaries, surviving members were annually assessed an equal share of the amounts paid out. Because payments made by all members were equal, an offer of membership in an assessment society amounted to an offer to participate in a pooling of dissimilar risks for a premium that did not reflect such dissimilarity. The result was unfortunate:

It was soon realized that benefits at lowest cost were obtainable when the majority of members were young. Young people, in the old society, with many older members, began to drop out when the assessments became frequent ... As the younger members dropped out ... the inevitable result was an abnormally high rate of assessment, and not infrequently a collapse of the organization. The attendant loss to those old members who had all their lives contributed to the benefits of others was disheartening and often tragic. (Magee 1958)

If there were competing societies, a newly formed society with only lower-age and thus lower-risk members would be most attractive. In more recent times, the experience of assessment societies was partly relived in the early years of health maintenance organizations, when the low average age of members resulted in costs that made the new organizations more competitive than older forms of health insurance. As might be expected, this advantage disappeared over the years. A more recent example is found in attempts to introduce community rating for health insurance. Under this approach, age and all other characteristics are not taken into account in setting rates. The predictable result is reduced participation by younger and healthier people. After New York adopted community rating for health insurance in 1993, "insurance rates for young people shot up by as much as 170% in the first year, prompting many of them to cancel policies." For one insurance company, the average age of policy owners increased by eight and a half years (Health Reform, the Sequel 1996). In each such situation, the fact that the structure did not recognize known risk differences, together with the organization's inability to mandate membership, caused a shift in membership to higher-risk individuals and, in the assessment society case, eventual failure.

Life Insurance Companies

The unfortunate experience of assessment societies demonstrates the need to reflect relative risk in the charges made by a voluntary organization intended to pool life insurance risks. The basic premise of assessment societies—that each member should share equally in assessments —did not offer an easy method of recognizing such differences in risk, even those caused by differences in age. The explicit recognition of age as a predictor of longevity characterizes the life insurance companies that thrived while the assessment societies were failing. These companies use a structure of level periodic payments and mathematically determined reserves to reflect the impact of age on risk.

Life insurance companies that use this structure might be organized as mutual companies or as stock companies, but in any case were in competition with one another for the voluntary business of individuals or groups. For both mutuals and stocks, the relationship with the individual customer is defined by a contract or policy. The policy contains conditions of coverage, as well as rates, or premiums, that must be paid initially and at subsequent intervals. Because each customer or policy owner enters into a separate contract, premiums can reflect differences in age or indeed in any other factor expected to affect the risk of death of the insured. Premiums can thus be designed to reflect the specific risks posed by each definable risk class.

Initially, life insurance companies primarily offered individual insurance, which pays a benefit only on the death of a specific individual (the insured). The policy owner might be the insured, another individual, or even a trust or other legal structure, but because this legal distinction does not normally affect the decision-making process, no generality is lost by restricting the consideration of individual insurance to the case where the policy owner is an individual.

In attempting to form a contract of insurance, a central concern is obviously the risk to be insured. Not all risks are suitable for insurance. In fact, insurance is usually limited to coverage that pays out on the occurrence of an insurable event. Generally speaking, five conditions must be met for an event to be considered insurable. First, it must result from an actuarial risk; in other words, it must involve uncertainty with respect to occurrence, timing, or severity. Second, this risk must display enough statistical regularity to allow its frequency of occurrence to be predicted with some degree of confidence. Third, the fact that the event has occurred must be definitely determinable. Fourth, the event must involve loss to one or more persons. Fifth, the person or persons suffering loss must not be in a position to influence the occurrence, timing, or severity of the event.

If a person has an insurable interest in an insured risk, this person is expected to suffer loss if the insured event occurs. Moreover, the insurer is expected be in a position to limit the insurance amount so that the person loses more than he or she would gain from the insurance benefit, thus reducing the chance of moral hazard. For life insurance, given the unacceptable course that moral hazard might take, the requirement of insurable interest has been inserted into state laws and regulations, and this is one of the primary reasons why a secondary market in life insurance policies has so far failed to develop in the United States.

Age and gender, the so-called census characteristics, are hard to conceal. They are, in effect, what information economists call common knowledge. In a competitive market, a decision to ignore common knowledge almost inevitably has unfavorable consequences for a participant in the market. If a life insurer chooses to lump together two or more risk classes that can be readily distinguished (for example, if a company chooses to use quinquennial age groupings to set premiums) competitors will almost certainly offer separate rates to the component classes. Lower-risk applicants will favor separated-rate competitors, and higher-risk applicants will choose the combined-class offering. In the end, the combined-class model will cover only the higher-risk end of the spectrum or be forced out of the market altogether.

This is a form of adverse selection, although it arises from actions of the insurer rather than those of the applicant. The applicant has more knowledge than is available to the insurer in making a contract offer, and the outcome is as expected: the quinquennial age contract will appeal to those near the higher end of the age bracket, and it will fail to attract anyone near the lower end of the bracket if single-age contracts are available. Unless differentiation has a significant cost, a firm acting alone cannot resist market pressure to fully reflect common knowledge.

Differentiating by age (and other items of common knowledge) is not enough to ensure the solidity of the life insurance enterprise. Lives considered for insurance differ with respect to health and other risk factors, and a rate structure to reflect such differences was instituted early in the history of the industry. This resulted in the division of each age group into standard and substandard rating classes. For more than a century and a half the standard class comprised over 90% of all offers of coverage in the United States and was intended to represent insured lives that had a reduced likelihood of survival relative to others in the age group. The standard class was thus considered relatively homogeneous, and a single rate was offered for each age. Over time, standard classes were further divided: in the 1920s, by the gender of the insured; in the 1970s and 1980s, into smoker and nonsmoker classes; and in the 1990s, into a set of preferred classes. These developments regarding the standard class are discussed later.

The substandard class, unlike the standard class, was highly heterogeneous: each age group included people who had recently suffered disease or possible symptoms of disease and those who pursued hazardous occupations or avocations, as well as those who in some other way presented an elevated risk of reduced longevity. Although various sources of risk could result in expected mortality above that of the standard class, the degree of elevation, and even its incidence over the years after issue of the policy, were not identical. The heterogeneity of the substandard class required its further subdivision to produce a rate structure that would be effective in the marketplace.

Because the substandard class represented a relatively small slice of the life insurance business, it was possible to treat each policy individually and produce, in effect, a custom rate for the proposed insured. The ingenious process that allowed such customization while nevertheless producing a rate structure that was internally consistent long ago became the industry standard (see chapter 4).

The information necessary to set substandard rates is not common knowledge in the information theory sense. Applicants start with more information about their health impairments and hazardous activities than does the insurer. Unless not permitted to do so by law or regulation, the insurer will normally seek to obtain this information, using questionnaires, queries to the potential insured's physician, medical or paramedical examinations, laboratory tests, and other sources. These procedures protect the insurer against adverse selection, and also may reveal information previously unknown to the applicant. From the insurer's perspective, the information, whether known to the applicant or not, helps assign the most appropriate rate, the rate based on the marginal cost of the contract to the insurer. However, from an information-economic point of view, the case where underwriting procedures are used to discover information already known to the applicant and the case where previously unknown information is unearthed are distinct situations. Prohibiting tests for previously unknown information would increase the difficulty in assuring that correct probabilities are used to develop rates, but preventing the insurer from obtaining information that the applicant already has could, in addition, cause information asymmetry and adverse selection. Analysis and comparison of these situations can be furthered by techniques associated with game theory.

Game theory is the study of transactions (broadly defined) in which two or more players choose strategies with the intent of maximizing their respective payoffs. Eric Rasmusen (1994) defined several examples he called insurance games to illustrate the application of game theory concepts to insurance. These examples belong to the category of "principal-agent" games. One set of players, the principals, tries to decide what sort of offer to make to another set of players, the agents. The agents are assumed to have more detailed information than do the principals. If the principals are taken to be insurers and the agents applicants for insurance, an economic game of this type becomes a quasi-realistic representation of the situation in which a life insurer does not have or is not permitted to use information, known to the applicant, about the prospective insured's life expectancy. One additional player is introduced into many games, including insurance games: Nature. Nature does not adopt strategies, but it does take actions at various points in the game. In the insurance games, it may, for example, move first and assign to each agent a set of survival probabilities. Alternatively, it may move after the contract has been agreed to, for example, by changing the survival probabilities.

Game theory gives precise definitions to some of the concepts we have introduced. An economic game has symmetric information if no player has information different from other players when he or she moves; otherwise it has asymmetric information (Rasmusen 1994, p. 45). Several kinds of games have asymmetric information; the two that most concern insurance are those that display moral hazard and those that display adverse selection. Moral hazard, as defined for game theory, occurs when the players begin with symmetric information and enter into a contract, after which one of the players (or Nature) makes a move unobserved by the other player. This is the situation faced by an insurer that issues an auto policy that pays a benefit if the car is stolen if the insured becomes careless about locking the car after being accepted for insurance.

More pertinent to this chapter are the insurance games displaying adverse selection. Here, in game-theoretic terms, Nature begins the game by giving each agent characteristics known to the agent but not to the principal. In these insurance games, it is usually assumed that there are two agents, one representing a "low" risk and one representing a "high" risk. Each agent is also assumed to have the same maximum indemnity amount—for example, the cost of the most expensive medical procedure. Game theory makes simplifying assumptions in order to highlight the essential aspects of the transactions being studied. One would not expect to make detailed numerical predictions of prices or other quantities with this sort of analysis. However, if the assumptions describe the essential characteristics of the market, it is possible to determine whether the market will actually be able to function effectively without intervention.

The game proceeds with the principal making an offer to each agent to enter a contract, specified by a coverage amount and a premium. If information about the agents' characteristics is supplied to the principal before the contracts are formed, and if the principal is allowed to classify the agents according to this information, the contracts offered to the low and high risks will have premium rates that reflect the relative expectations of claims. Moreover, Cummins et al. (1982) show that the amount of coverage purchased by both low- and high-risk agents will be the maximum indemnity amount.

If, on the other hand, the contracts are entered into with the agents having more relevant information than do the principals (for example, the low- and high-risk agents know their risk level, but the principals do not), and if the principals settle on their pricing strategies without taking account of the reaction that the other principals may have to their strategy choices, Cummins et al. show that the resulting adverse selection precludes a stable market. One might expect that all the principals would simply offer a contract with the weighted average premium. This offer would result in an equilibrium if all insurers had perfect foresight about the consequences of their strategic choices, but by assumption, the insurers are "myopic" and do not anticipate competitors' reactions. Thus, one of the insurers may be expected to offer a new contract, which is preferred to the would-be equilibrium contract by low-risk applicants but not by high-risk applicants. Unfortunately, once the second contract is offered, the original contract becomes unprofitable and is withdrawn. Then, high-risk applicants are forced to purchase the new contract, and that, too, will become unprofitable. In the end, no contract can remain profitable, so all insurers will withdraw from the market.

A potentially workable alternative strategy is to offer two contracts, one that will be preferred by low-risk applicants and another that will be preferred by high-risk applicants. Under some circumstances, this strategy is successful. The result is a *self-selection*, or *separating, equilibrium* in the market. Effectively, the market has found a way to introduce the hidden information into an equilibrium price structure through the choices made by the agents. Unfortunately, at this equilibrium the higher-risk applicants pay as much as they would pay in a market without adverse selection (where their true risk was known and priced), and the lower-risk applicants pay *more* than they would in a full-information market—an unequivocal welfare loss has thus occurred.

Unfortunately, the usual analysis of games with adverse selection makes some assumptions that may not apply to life insurance. First, the maximum indemnity amount is hard to determine for life insurance. The value of a car or a building can be ascertained and used to determine the maximum amount of indemnification to be offered, but for life insurance, the needs range widely and are hard to quantify. The insurer may be far more flexible about the amounts offered on a given life, making the game theory analysis harder to apply.

The assumption that insurers choose their strategies without taking account of possible reactions of their competitors can also be challenged. Equilibria formed under this assumption are called Nash equilibria after John Nash, the 1994 Nobel laureate in economics. Other conditions leading to other equilibria can be defined. However, the life insurance market in the United States is highly fragmented, despite important mergers in the 1980s and 1990s. More than 1500 companies compete in this market, and over 200 have significant presence.

Although the behavior of principals under a Nash equilibrium was described as myopic, it is not unusual to see life insurers react to the current marketplace without considering countermoves. Actuarial students have long referred to this pricing philosophy as "take off a nickel." Specifically, each insurer tends to define a peer group that it tracks. Since the pricing process, including regulatory filing, takes from two to nine months, it is difficult to respond to current activity of the peer group, much less to potential countermoves to a pricing change.

For a number of reasons that were not incorporated into the insurance games just described, achieving a pooling equilibrium in the face of adverse selection is harder in a life insurance market than in a market for other forms of insurance. Difficulty specifying the appropriate amount of indemnification is the first problem. Life insurance may be purchased for many reasons. The most commonly referenced is the need to replace the income stream of an individual who is counted on to produce a salary or other earnings that will terminate with his or her death. Another reason is the need to hedge the outcome of a contract in which significant amounts of money are promised for future services, as may be the case with athletes or entertainers. Funds are also needed to liquify assets, such as small businesses, in case one of several owners dies, and to provide for tax bills and other expenses that may occur at death. These needs vary, and the amount of life insurance needed to indemnify each of these diverse risks varies not only with the individual situation, but with the degree of risk aversion of those indemnified.

It is difficult to determine a weighted average when the benefit amounts that may be requested vary widely. Presumably, higher-risk applicants would want more coverage at any given price, thus inserting an additional layer of adverse selection. This difficulty is aggravated by other factors. For instance, the distribution of high-risk applicants among insurers may not be uniform. Higher-risk applicants could be clustered geographically or socioeconomically so that certain firms are more likely than others to receive applications from this group. During the early years of the AIDS epidemic, it was apparent that certain firms received an overabundance of applications from heavily affected groups, perhaps based on word of mouth about their underwriting practices.

These difficulties are compounded by the fact that life insurance involves a high degree of leverage and is heavily dependent on the time value of money. For example, at some ages a $1,000 annual premium can buy more than one million dollars of life insurance coverage. The present value at 5% interest of this benefit is only $231,000 if death occurs thirty years from now, compared with $952,000 if it occurs one year from now. Thus, especially if the higher-risk group has a much higher annual probability of death, even a small admixture of higher risks can raise the cost of coverage substantially for an insurer, and, if it cannot be sure its competitors will all receive a similar admixture, it may choose not to participate in the market. These factors—difficulty determining indemnification needs, potential clustering, and the high degree of leverage—taken together make a pooling equilibrium hard to achieve for life insurance.

Another assumption implicit in the insurance games is that information about survival probabilities can be obtained by the insurer without cost. In fact, the risk-classification process has important costs. First, and in some contexts most important, is the opportunity cost represented by applicants deciding not to consider a contract that requires medical examinations or other forms of sometimes unpleasant information gathering. Establishment of testing requirements may in itself have a positive selective effect, but invasive testing will also cause an insurer to miss out on lower-risk applicants with a low tolerance for such tests.

More generally recognized is that underwriting itself has a cost. Medical and paramedical examinations, laboratory tests on blood and urine, as well as reports obtained from personal physicians, departments of motor vehicles, and credit agencies each have a cost, and analysis of additional data requires time and effort on the part of the home office underwriter. Insurers must limit the average cost of underwriting a case to the average amount provided for this purpose in pricing the policy. To decide which tests to use, insurers rely on studies of protective value. The protective value of a test is the net cost savings produced by the use of the test, i.e., the reduction of mortality cost minus the cost of the test.

Defined in this way, it is easy to see that the protective value of a test will increase with the amount of insurance applied for. This leads many insurers to set a nonmedical limit. Policies with face amounts at or below the nonmedical limit are not subjected to medical underwriting at all. Obviously, such policies are priced differently from medically underwritten ones.

A significant incidence of adverse selection was experienced in conjunction with the AIDS epidemic by some companies, but not others, on policies written for exactly the nonmedical limit. From a game theoretic point of view, adverse selection may be explained by signaling (Rasmusen 1994, pp. 249–271). Since applications for nonmedical policies can be declined, an application for a $99,999 policy can be viewed as a signal that the applicant has reasons for avoiding medical underwriting. Applicants who had something to hide could be expected to avoid such signals. On the other hand, most people purchase insurance in round amounts, and applications for $100,000 policies are very common, regardless of the existence of nonmedical limits. Thus, an application for a $100,000 policy would not be seen as a signal, even if this was the nonmedical limit. In fact, companies that sold $100,000 policies on a nonmedical basis had very heavy early claims compared with those that required medical underwriting beginning with that amount.

Protective value is important in insurers' decisions about which tests to request. If a test can be requested only if other indications strongly point to a need for the information, it will often be required. However, if a test must be given to every applicant to be effective, its cost must fit into the relatively limited amount allotted to the underwriting of every policy. Tests that are frequently part of the normal underwriting profile include (at the time of writing) tests for HIV, cotinine tests for smoking, measurements of cholesterol and the high-density lipoprotein ratio, and liver function tests. At certain ages, prostate-specific antigen measurement may be required for men, and electrocardiograms may be required for higher insurance amounts (the threshold may depend on the age and gender of the applicant).

Sufficient loads to pay for such a test profile are commonly built into fully underwritten policies. Recently, several insurers substituted oral fluid tests for blood tests for lower face amounts (perhaps up to $500,000 or more), mainly to streamline the underwriting and issuing process and to avoid the opportunity cost. Protective value studies may support such actions, since expected mortality is still reduced, although not as much as with full blood tests, and the cost of the test is much lower.

One additional source of adverse selection should be mentioned: a secondary market.

As mentioned, until recently there was no secondary market for life insurance in the United States. During the AIDS epidemic of the early 1990s, a number of policy owners found themselves holding life insurance policies purchased prior to the epidemic, while they, at the same time, faced mounting medical bills. In response to this situation, a number of "viatical" organizations arose. The viaticals attempted to provide a secondary market through bundling and securitizing life insurance policies covering AIDS victims and others with terminal illnesses. In the late 1990s and early 2000s, similar organizations also attempted to securitize life insurance policies belonging to older persons under the rubric "senior settlements." Both viaticals and senior settlement organizations recognized the possibility of adverse selection against them and thus employed a form of "reverse underwriting" to ensure against unwonted longevity.

An important side-effect of viaticals and senior settlements on the life insurance market is increased incentive for applicants with impairments to hide this information from the insurer, since the policy, if issued, could provide an immediate payout to the applicant him- or herself far in excess of the initial premium. In other words, a secondary market would likely increase the likelihood of adverse selection and even misrepresentation by life insurance applicants. It would also increase the protective value of tests (genetic tests might, for example, become worthwhile from a protective-value point of view) and induce insurers to increase the level of underwriting for all sizes and types of policies. It could well eliminate or marginalize nonmedical, simplified- and guaranteed-issue policies sold on an individual basis. Current viatical and senior settlement initiatives have not engendered an overly enthusiastic response, so this is, for the moment, only a theoretical concern.

Group and Social Insurance

The process of forming contracts depends, of course, on the nature and relationship of the contracting parties. Voluntary individual insurance, under which contracts designed by insurers without significant constraint are offered to the public, is only one of several relationship structures that could be employed. Two of the most important alternatives are social insurance and group insurance.

Under social insurance, the insurer is the government; the risk insured may be a person's life, health, or retirement income; and premiums (often designated as taxes) are paid either by the insured or by his or her employer. Social insurance is generally mandatory (coverage is required by law) although in a few instances government provides insurance for which participation is not required. If coverage is not mandatory, or if it is provided as an alternative to the private market, social insurance can be subject to adverse selection. This has caused difficulties for many state-run assigned risk pools for automobile insurance.

Mandatory social insurance is established by law, not by contract. No underwriting is required since coverage is provided to all who are eligible. Mandatory health insurance is subject to moral hazard and rent seeking by providers. Rent is formally defined as "that part of a person's or firm's income which is above the minimum amount necessary to keep that person or firm in its given occupation" (Henderson and Quandt 1971, p. 121). It is also necessary to introduce artificial allocation mechanisms such as queueing. In contrast, mandatory life insurance is rarely offered in meaningful amounts because of difficulty determining indemnification needs. Its beneficial aspects of mandatory participation would be lost if the amount of coverage were discretionary, but a uniform flat benefit, such as was offered with Social Security from the beginning of that program, must either be useless to many or an unaffordable windfall to most.

Group insurance provides coverage for risks pertaining to a group of individual participants under a single contract issued to a sponsor. Typically, the sponsor is the employer of the participants, although group-type coverage may be used in other contexts. Group insurance is achieved through a voluntary contract between the sponsor and the insurer. Participants are not parties to the contract itself, although a subsidiary arrangement may exist between the participant and the sponsor or insurer that creates legal rights. Participation in group insurance may be mandatory or voluntary, but in the latter case some minimum level of participation is usually required by the insurer as a condition of the contract. If the group is large enough, this condition obviates some of the difficulties discussed in this chapter and allows a premium to be set based on characteristics of the group, rather than on characteristics of each participant. In most cases, the premium can be revised periodically, often annually.

This feature also eliminates concerns that are important for other types of insurance. Underwriting for group contracts involves consideration of characteristics of the group, rather than of individual members of the group, for the most part. For example, the rate paid by the contract holder may depend on the nature of the work done by participants and on the distribution of ages and genders of the participants but rarely on health or hazardous avocations of individual members.

In some cases, individual underwriting is applied to members of the group if they have disproportionately large benefits. Group underwriting may be applied to contracts that are legally structured as individual policies. This is the case, for example, with corporate-owned life insurance, in which a company insures a number of usually high-level employees using individual policies. Groups are subject to another form of risk that does not affect individuals—concentration or accumulation risk. As concerns about terrorism arose in the early years of the new millennium, underwriting for concentration risk became important to group insurers. For terrorism, the concern is physical concentration, say of employees in a single high-rise building, but concentration risk may also have been present during the AIDS epidemic, even without physical proximity at work.

Provisions for Unobserved Relative Risk—The Emergence of Preferred Classes

One advantage attributed to market-based life insurance is the likelihood that premiums in a competitive marketplace will be lower than can be arranged by other mechanisms. If the marketplace can be assumed to be competitive, traditional microeconomics would say that optimal performance would occur when prices of the product are based on its marginal cost.

The most important part of the marginal cost is the cost of the life insurance benefit itself. Thus, for this marketplace to operate optimally, insurers have to know about anything that might affect survival probabilities, not only currently observable conditions such as illness and hazardous occupations, avocations or lifestyle, but other evidence that helps assess the risk of future illnesses or hazards, if these illnesses and hazards are likely to affect life expectancy.

Dramatic demonstrations of the relationship of risk assessment and premium optimality occurred from time to time as new underwriting information or tests became available and were applied by the industry. For example, premium distinctions based on gender appeared in the 1920s as the need for coverage for women began to emerge with women's greater role in business and industry. Over the next eighty years the longevity of women improved relatively faster than that of similar-age men. The marketplace reacted to this and produced female rates that tend to be 30% to 40% lower than male rates.

In the late 1960s and 1970s, studies on the health impact of smoking led to distinctions in premiums for smokers and nonsmokers. Companies that were slow to introduce these distinctions in their pricing found themselves taking on a more than proportionate share of smokers as standard risks, and their financial results suffered noticeably.

Introduction of preferred underwriting in the late 1980s and early 1990s provides another example of the tendency of the life insurance market to move to a new equilibrium involving lower overall cost when new underwriting techniques become available. Preferred underwriting is a term for the division of the traditional standard class into subclasses based on refined classification. Before this development, all "healthy" individuals of the same age, gender, and smoking history were grouped

Table 3.1
Ten-Year Level Premium Term (typical rate per $1,000, male, age 45, non-smoker, $250,000 face amount of insurance)

	Best preferred class	"Standard" class
1997	$1.67	$3.08
1992	2.26 (25%)	3.10 (1%)
1990	2.64 (37%)	3.03 (−2%)

Source: Dicke 1998, figure 14.

together into one large standard class. From 90% to 95% of life insurance offers were made on the standard basis. Only insureds with actual sickness or hazard, or significant estimable risk of future illness, were placed in substandard classes. The new preferred classes tried to estimate the relative risk of death due to future illness or trauma by looking at things such as cholesterol levels, driving records, and liver function tests (the last being, among other things, a way to gauge alcohol abuse), as well as cotinine tests for tobacco use that could verify statements made by the applicant.

When preferred underwriting was introduced, it was commonly believed that any decrease in the cost of insurance for those satisfying the new, more stringent requirements would be made up for by correspondingly higher premiums paid by those relegated to the residual standard class. That was not what happened, at least not in every case. From 1991 to 1996, premiums for preferred classes fell by as much as 35%, a decrease that has continued at a slower pace to the present day. But, despite such expectations, for some companies the standard class rate did not increase significantly. Table 3.1 shows this effect in premiums charged for coverage of a forty-five-year-old standard-class male by a representative company during that period of time (Dicke 1998, figure 14).

What can explain the observed result: the premium for preferred risks carved out from the standard class falling significantly, while premiums for the rest of the risks that would also have been standard remain stable? One possible answer looks to the same factors that were cited above to show why it is difficult to achieve a pooling equilibrium among substandard classes. These factors were inability to define indemnification needs, potential clustering of higher-risk applicants, and the high degree of leverage available in life insurance. The standard class had been thought to be homogeneous, but new testing technology showed it to be quite heterogeneous; not to the degree of substandard classes, but enough to cause difficulties in achieving a pooling equilibrium. In an environment of uncertainty about the average level of risk represented by the standard class, the market demanded a risk premium. When the uncertainty was reduced by refined classification, none of the separate rates required this premium, and the aggregate rate charged was reduced.

The impact of the introduction of preferred underwriting in the 1990s on the price of life insurance, as well as effects experienced in connection with earlier introduction of gender and smoking differentials, indicate that underwriting improvements may lead to a decreased overall price of life insurance to the public. This is in fact what would be predicted by microeconomic theory. The industry's ability to judge more accurately the marginal cost of coverage allows the market to demand a risk premium of a lower amount.

Moreover, ability to assess the risk more accurately allows for more price competition among insurers. Life insurers, insofar as they pursue economic advantage for themselves and their owners, would be expected to have no preference for an insured at one risk level over an insured at another risk level, provided that the premium properly covers the expected cost. When this condition does not hold, individual companies may try to find some surrogate for underwriting. For example, a company may attempt to market only in areas that are thought to contain a larger proportion of lower-risk individuals than other areas. A company competing in a marketplace that provides coverage to a variety of risks for the same premium will succeed to the degree that it is able to sign up more favorable risks. On the other hand, if all risks are priced according to the marginal cost represented by the present value of future expected claims, every insured represents the same profit potential for every insurer. An insurer's strategy no longer involves finding market segments that are likely to be more profitable, but rather trying by traditional competitive means—lower prices and better service—to attract as many customers as possible at each risk level. This increased competition in all segments is likely to produce lower overall costs and better overall service.

Interventions to Reduce Impact on Higher-Risk Individuals

Whereas extensions of underwriting to new criteria will produce a more optimal overall pricing structure and thus a lower cost of insurance to society as a whole, individuals may find life insurance discouragingly expensive if they should fall into classes with very high risk. This did not emerge as a significant problem relative to substandard classes that had been used for many years, perhaps because individuals who were or recently had been ill or who recognized that they lived, worked, or played in hazardous circumstances were not inclined to dispute the premiums. The situation is different, however, when the possibility of using genetic tests for underwriting is raised.

To a life insurer, a test for genetic abnormalities looks in many ways like any of the other underwriting tools that it has traditionally used to place potential insureds in the proper risk class. Genetic conditions may imply reduced expectations of longevity and thus change the marginal cost of providing coverage on the individual. On the other hand, genetic tests may indicate actions that can be taken to achieve greater longevity. For example, with hemochromatosis, regular blood transfusions can control the potentially lethal build-up of iron in internal organs. Evidence that such actions have been taken reduces the marginal cost of life insurance coverage.

To the applicant, on the other hand, genetic information may seem different from information derived from other medical tests that predict longevity. An individual may think that he or she can reduce cholesterol level and thereby change the likelihood of early death from that cause; however, a person with certain genetic conditions (including some forms of elevated cholesterol level) cannot at present change those conditions by an action that he or she might take. Moreover, by determining whether a deleterious gene is present, genetic tests may abruptly change longevity expectations. For example, in the case of Huntington disease, the presence of a particular mutation means development of clinical disease is inevitable, most often in the thirties or forties, with death occurring in another ten to twenty years. The absence of that alteration indicates the likelihood of a normal life span.

For conditions such as Huntington disease, at-risk individuals applying for life insurance may provide favorable results of genetic tests to obtain standard or preferred rates. Life insurers normally accept such information and use it to determine appropriate rates. In fact, they want access to genetic test results that are known to the applicant. Without assurance that results known to the applicant will be available to underwriters, insurers would have to assume that adverse selection will occur and cause significant losses. On the other hand, insurers, at least at present, are almost always willing to forego the right to require genetic tests for applicants who have not previously taken them. They obtain information from family histories that provide some of the same insights that could be expected from genetic tests, although in the case of such conditions as Huntington disease, the outcome of genetic tests can allow a decreased premium. But the definitiveness of the test for Huntington disease is unusual; in fact, at present few genetic tests have sufficient predictive ability to justify their fairly high cost. Thus, life insurers may be willing to leave the choice of whether to undergo a genetic test to applicants as long as results of any test undergone are made available to the company.

This approach appears on the surface to preserve the status quo for both life insurers and applicants. However, it has the disadvantage of discouraging those at risk for certain potentially ameliorable genetic conditions from having the appropriate test, and it may discourage others from taking part in research involving genetic tests. The individual at risk for a gene-based condition may be concerned that an unfavorable result would preclude qualifying for some form of insurance coverage. Thus, the test itself may be seen as a source of potential loss.

Many suggestions have been made for assisting individuals who face this circumstance. Most of them involve either direct or indirect subsidies to the individual. For example, it is often proposed that insurers be banned by law or regulation from acquiring or using information developed through genetic tests. From an economic point of view, this produces a subsidy because the individual at high risk is provided coverage at standard rates. If the reinsurer can accurately determine the number of high-risk individuals in a specific underwriting class, the impact is likely to be an increase in rates applicable to that class to cover the higher expected rate of claims. As discussed, difficulty determining indemnification needs, the possibility of clustering, and the high leverage associated with life insurance imply that the insurer will have to add a risk premium as well as the expected additional claim cost to the price of coverage. In any case, if the market reaches equilibrium at all, the result is a subsidy in the form of lower rates for high-risk individuals, with the subsidy in this case being paid for by other members of the risk class.

Three questions must be asked about a proposed subsidy: is it justified and for whom, how large should it be, and who will be responsible for paying its cost? Looked at this way, numerous alternative choices emerge. Limiting availability of certain information is only one, and involves a subsidy of an unlimited amount to those at higher risk, paid for by other policy owners who participate in such market.

Alternatively, the subsidy could be provided by the government. The government, of course, would have to obtain funds from some source: general revenues (which in turn are paid for by taxpayers), a special tax on insurers, or even more intricate mechanisms. One advantage of the government approach is that it could be designed in such a way as to reduce or eliminate the risk premiums that insurers may find it necessary to charge. If a government subsidy is paid directly to an affected individual to allow the purchase of coverage at the appropriate risk-adjusted premium, the efficiency of the insurance mechanism will not be compromised, although overall efficiency of the economy may be affected. If the cost is allocated back to insurers through a special tax, the cost of coverage will be increased by the expected tax, but the uncertainty, and thus the risk premium, might not appear. Direct payments to affected parties by the government do, however, have drawbacks. For example, the recipient would have to provide sensitive information to the government, and the entire process might be considered unduly intrusive.

Mechanisms have been suggested that would be administered by the insurers collectively without government involvement. Several proposals were made for implementing such risk-adjustment mechanisms in the health insurance arena. In effect, each insurer provides coverage at standard rates, but receives payments for higher-risk individuals it covers. The extra cost of such coverage is transferred to a pool funded by insurers on a basis proportional to some measure, such as overall market share. The idea is to provide subsidies the cost of which can be shared equitably among insurers and recouped through increased premiums paid by policy holders. Unfortunately, the administrative complexities of such arrangements can be daunting.

An interesting alternative eliminates the need for subsidy altogether. Known as testing insurance, it is based on the observation that testing itself (for genetic or other conditions with similar effect) could satisfy the requirements of being an insurable event. A test clearly does involve uncertainty, and its outcome is definitely determinable and may have undesirable economic consequences for a person who cannot know or control the outcome. Testing insurance would indemnify loss caused by the test. Before the test is taken, a premium is paid to the insurer providing testing coverage. If the test result is favorable, no further payments are made. If the test has an unfavorable outcome, a benefit is paid to the individual sufficient to indemnify the loss incurred by taking the test. For example, an unfavorable genetic test would result in a payment sufficient to allow the immediate purchase of a specified amount of life and health insurance.

Because statistical regularity is not established and because the cost of providing the benefit is not known with sufficient accuracy, testing insurance is only an academic idea at present. To determine the economic viability of the idea for a specific genetic test, the test would have to be given to a statistically significant number of persons, and statistics on the outcomes would have to be made available to insurers interested in providing testing insurance coverage. Also, mortality and morbidity connected with the condition tested for would have to be studied to estimate the value of the benefit.

One attractive possibility, if reasonably priced testing were available, would be to have the premium for testing insurance added to the price of the test itself. It could be argued that the firm that offers the genetic tests has a responsibility to provide this sort of coverage for subjects taking the test.

At our current state of knowledge, only for a few gene-based conditions can the risk of future impairment be determined with sufficient accuracy to allow life insurance premiums covering such risks to be set with confidence. Moreover, the cost of tests for these conditions remains high relative to amounts that insurers can allocate to pay for them. For these reasons, the social benefit in terms of decreased overall cost of life insurance that would result from genetic testing at the current level of knowledge is probably insufficient to warrant insurers' routine use of these tests.

This may not always be the case. Preferred underwriting segments the standard class mainly by using criteria that indicate elevated risk of death due to trauma or cardiovascular conditions. If tests become available that are able to differentiate risk levels for the more common cancers, their potential economic benefit would be great. Also, as these tests become better able to predict potentially life-shortening conditions, the temptation to hide negative outcomes will increase, unless deception can be discovered during underwriting, presumably by requiring such tests.

It is clear, however, that to use these tests, whether to offer even lower preferred rates or to ward off adverse selection, consideration must be given to moderating the effect on individuals. Economic analysis can be a valuable tool in choosing the method of amelioration that helps individuals most affected, while allowing the market mechanism to operate with sufficient freedom to produce optimal social results.

Conclusion

Traditional economic analysis based on supply and demand and indifference curves, now augmented by newer analysis of information economics, is a valuable tool for understanding the life insurance marketplace. This marketplace has characteristics specific to it, and some of the traditional analysis applied to property-casualty and health risks must be modified when dealing with life insurance. Because the industry has been delivering increased coverage for reduced premiums over two centuries in the United States in a market where benefits are regulated lightly and prices not at all, it is reasonable to suggest that careful economic analysis should precede any fundamental change. Such analysis may be useful not just to ensure optimal benefit to society as a whole, but also to weigh, and even invent, approaches that can assist those disadvantaged by the workings of the system while not unduly reducing the efficiency of the market.

References

Cummins, B. D. et al., Risk Classification in Life Insurance. Hingham, MA: Kluwer-Nijhoff (1982).

Dicke, A. A., "The Preferred Underwriting Revolution: Impact on the Life

Insurance Market," The Ross-Huebner-McCahan lecture, Nov. 18, 1997. Philadelphia: University of Pennsylvania (1998).

"Health Reform, the Sequel," Investor's Business Daily, March 25, 1996.

Henderson, J. N. and Quandt, R. E., Microeconomic Theory: A Mathematical Approach, 2d ed. New York: McGraw-Hill (1971).

Magee, J. H., Life Insurance, 3d ed. Homewood, IL: Richard D. Irwin (1958).

Rasmusen, E., Games and Information: An Introduction to Game Theory, 2d ed. Cambridge, MA: Blackwell (1994).

4

Medical Underwriting

Robert K. Gleeson

Many Americans have a small amount of life insurance as a benefit of employment; however, it is seldom sufficient to provide for total family protection, college education, or business coverage in the event of premature death. To cover these financial needs people buy individually underwritten life insurance from the private market in different amounts and at different times throughout their life.

People seeking this protection are free to choose when to buy, what to buy, and how much to pay for coverage. They can buy when they are young and healthy, or wait until middle age hoping their health will stay good, or they can buy at a higher premium if they develop a chronic illness. Based on their total financial portfolio, moneys available, and coverage needs, they can choose products ranging from an inexpensive term insurance product to a high cash value (whole life) product and everything in between. More than 1,500 companies compete aggressively to sell life insurance to meet these different needs.

The private life insurance system provides an important financial safety net, but it is entirely voluntary and unsubsidized. An individual life insurance policy is, in effect, a commercial transaction in which the insurer agrees to pay a specified death benefit in exchange for payment of a premium proportional to the mortality risk assumed by the insurer. (Nowlan 2002)

The one characteristic common to all individual life insurance products is transfer of the financial loss caused by unexpected death to the life insurance company. The real product is payment of the death benefit regardless of when that death occurs during the lifetime of the product. The death benefit for each individual far exceeds annual and cumulative premiums plus earnings for several years, particularly for young applicants.

To offer this financial protection, the company must to be able to identify and distinguish the risks each applicant poses, assess these risks, charge the appropriate premium to cover the risks, and invest wisely so that sufficient moneys exist to pay all present and future claims. Different groups of insureds with different life expectancies must be distinct based on real differences in mortality expectation. Industry credibility and financial stability require that these mortality and pricing differences be identifiable, equitable, and accurate.

Life expectancy varies by age, gender, medical and family histories, avocation, and lifestyle. Applicants for life insurance have different medical histories and risk factors for future disease that affect life expectancy. The purpose of any risk-selection or underwriting process is to place applicants into distinct groups that have similar expectations of life or risk of death at any time interval. Each group is charged a premium sufficient to cover costs associated with its expected rate of death. Insureds in each group have the same expectation of life (risk of death), pay equally, and are self-supporting. No group or person unfairly subsidizes any other group.

Applicants without a history of a diagnosed disease, adverse medical history, or significant risk factor are usually grouped in a large best class and considered to have standard mortality. Some companies further separate standard individuals by cardiovascular risk factor assessment into preferred or select classes. Insureds who are offered preferred life insurance policies have very low mortality and will pay the lowest rates.

Applicants may also have had or currently have almost every possible medical condition or disease, laboratory or radiological test result, or medical treatment. Those with different diseases or medical conditions can be grouped into risk categories with similar expectation of life and risk of premature death. For example, a person with a coronary artery disease risk and a diabetic patient both have double the expected annual mortality; both would pay the same premium because they share the same life expectancy.

The primary task of an underwriter is to assess life expectancy based on medical, occupational, and avocational factors significant to life expectancy. It is vital that the insurer have a full understanding, and particularly the same knowledge, as the applicant in order to assess accurately that risk equitably.

Life insurers are in business to sell life insurance. They are under intense competitive pressure to underwrite accurately and price the product attractively. This means that medical underwriters must identify a group with very favorable mortality to receive the lowest pricing and select the best applicants who have a given disease. Properly priced, rated business with less than standard mortality is as good (profitable) as nonrated business. Insurers make every possible attempt to put every applicant into the most favorable risk category at the best price.

Risk Selection in a Regulated and Competitive Environment

Different companies have different business models, target markets, investment philosophies, and mortality goals. Some sell only term insurance priced for a younger market, whereas others specialize in permanent cash value life insurance to more affluent markets. Some companies primarily sell policies in the $25,000 range and others sell very large policies averaging a million dollars. Some companies target preferred risks, whereas others specialize in underwriting impaired lives. Some companies price their product assuming a high lapse rate and others assume their products will stay in force for decades. Some companies want to have the lowest mortality in the industry and others want to run in the middle of the pack.

This competitive free market environment gives consumers opportunities to obtain many offers and prices for their insurance needs even if they have a disease or significant risk factor. Life insurance companies maintain medical staffs and underwriting specialists to find an edge in mortality gains that are translated as lower prices and wider availability to the consumer. These staffs evaluate the mortality impact of advances in medical knowledge, disease treatment, and test development. When an applicant with a known disease or test result applies for insurance, the medical underwriter must correctly identify and assess the risk and its significance. This applies whether the testing technology is as old as a basic blood count or as new as a DNA-based test. This free market process ensures that some companies are always on the leading edge of aggressive underwriting, and customers can get the best price for their life insurance needs regardless of their medical condition.

Individual life insurance is a carefully regulated product. In the United States, life insurance is primarily regulated by states. States require that insurance companies maintain adequate reserves to pay all future claims and that the application and underwriting processes are fair. The National Association of Insurance Commissioners (NAIC) brings loose coordination to the process. "Most states have laws that provide that life insurance companies may not discriminate unfairly among individuals of the same class and with equal expectation of life in premiums, policy terms, benefit, or dividend. State laws also prohibit unfair discrimination because of sex, marital status, race, religion, or national origin" (Black and Skipper 1994, p. 683).

Risk selection distinguishes private free market life insurance from government programs. Government insurance programs treat all individuals identically without regard to individual needs, health status, or contribution to the pool. The participation, premiums, and benefits are all mandated and apply equally to everyone regardless of their likelihood of needing or receiving the benefit. For example, almost all working Americans are required to participate in Social Security, and the same deductions are made from every paycheck regardless of the age of the applicant and likelihood for future benefits. By design, the Social Security system currently provides very limited death benefits but generous survivor (spouse and minor children) benefits.

The private free market individual life insurance system permits an applicant to decide when, if ever, to buy a policy and to determine the amount of coverage based on individual and changing personal financial needs. The process of risk selection or underwriting makes this choice possible and equitable.

Life Expectancy

People in any large group will die at a predictable rate. This is true for large groups totally free of disease as well as for those with a known disease or other risk factors. A group of young adults has an expected annual death rate that is substantially lower than that for an elderly group. A group of sixty-five-year-old marathoners has a much lower mortality than a group of sixty-five-year-olds in a cardiac rehabilitation program.

A group of 10,000 healthy twenty-year-old women has an expected life span to age eighty. Unfortunately, accidents and catastrophic illnesses take their toll in every year of life, and one of the twenty-year-olds will not see her twenty-first birthday. Half of the original group will be alive at age eighty, and a few of them will die before age eighty-one. A few of the 5,000 who reach eighty years will live to become truly old. In fact, about as many people in this group will live past age 100 as die before age thirty.

The *Vital Statistics of the United States* is based on a study of the entire population (Vital Statistics, 2003). Table 4.1 shows the number of years of life remaining at any given age and improvements in mortality that occurred during the past century. For example, a five-year-old girl has a life expectancy of five + seventy-five years, or age eighty. This is longer than a newborn because of the high death rate of newborns. The table shows that the life expectancy of a thirty-year-old man is 45.7 more years for a total of 75.7 years, whereas the life expectancy of a sixty-five-year-old man is 16.1 more years for a total of 81.7 years. The message is that you have to live to sixty-five before you can live to eighty.

Table 4.1 includes the entire population. At every age, it includes the large group of healthy individuals, a group with underlying medical conditions or risk factors, a small group with a chronic illness, and a very small group with serious illness.

These same data can be expressed as the number of deaths in each age group from a starting population of 100,000 people. Table 4.2 shows the expected deaths in five-year intervals for the general population. The mortality rate for the first year of life is twenty-five times higher than the annual rate for children age one to nine (Vital Statistics 2003). It is lowest in the preteen and early teen years but increases at age sixteen when teenagers begin to drive. From age thirty onward, a continuous and steady increase is seen in the mortality curve of nearly 10% per year from age forty to eighty.

This information is most useful to an actuary when the information is stated as deaths per 1,000 people of a given age and gender per year. Actuaries express their numbers as deaths per 1,000 in any given year or time interval. Insurers work with the number of expected deaths per year in a given population by age and gender similar to those of the Vital Statistics data. Table 4.3 shows information for the general population

Table 4.1
Average Number of Years of Life Remaining for the United States Population

Age (yrs)	Female			Male		
	1900–1902	1949–1951	1999	1900–1902	1949–1951	1999
0	50.70	70.96	79.4	47.88	65.47	73.9
1	56.10	71.84	78.9	54.35	66.73	73.5
5	55.80	68.21	75.0	54.22	63.12	69.6
10	51.94	63.38	70.1	50.39	58.35	64.7
15	47.60	58.52	65.1	46.06	53.56	59.8
20	43.60	53.73	60.2	42.03	48.92	55.0
25	39.92	48.99	55.4	38.38	44.36	50.4
30	36.30	44.28	50.5	34.76	39.78	45.7
35	32.71	39.63	45.7	31.19	35.23	41.1
40	29.08	35.06	41.0	27.65	30.79	36.5
45	25.44	30.64	36.3	24.14	26.55	32.0
50	21.84	26.40	31.7	20.70	22.59	27.7
55	18.39	22.33	27.3	17.38	18.96	23.5
60	15.21	18.50	23.1	14.33	15.68	19.6
65	12.22	14.95	19.1	11.50	12.74	16.1
70	9.59	11.71	15.4	9.02	10.11	12.8
75	7.34	8.94	12.1	6.84	7.83	10.0
80	5.51	6.67	9.1	5.11	5.94	7.5
85	4.12	4.90	6.6	3.82	4.41	5.5
90	3.04	3.54	4.8	2.86	3.30	4.1
95	2.24	2.57	3.5	2.13	2.49	3.0
100	1.61	1.93	2.7	1.55	1.92	2.4

Source: U.S. Department of Health and Human Services, National Vital Statistics Reports, vol. 50, no. 6, p. 11 (Table 11), March 21, 2002.

Table 4.2
Abridged Life Table for the Total Population: United States, 1999

Age (yrs)	Number living at beginning of age interval	Number dying during age interval	Life expectancy at beginning of age interval
0–1	100,000	706	76.7
1–5	99,294	137	76.3
5–10	99,157	87	72.4
10–15	99,070	104	67.4
15–20	98,966	345	62.5
20–25	98,621	461	57.7
25–30	98,160	476	53.0
30–35	97,684	575	48.2
35–40	97,109	788	43.5
40–45	96,321	1,131	38.8
45–50	95,190	1,669	34.3
50–55	93,521	2,398	29.8
55–60	91,123	3,670	25.5
60–65	87,453	5,433	21.5
65–70	82,020	7,736	17.7
70–75	74,284	10,485	14.3
75–80	63,799	13,273	11.2
80–85	50,526	16,059	8.5
85–90	34,467	16,022	6.3
90–95	18,445	11,424	4.6
95–100	7,021	5,326	3.4
100+	1,695	1,695	2.6

Source: U.S. Department of Health and Human Services, National Vital Statistics Reports, vol. 50, no. 6, p. 38, March 21, 2002.

Table 4.3
Number of Deaths per 1,000 Lives

Age (yrs)	Female		Male	
	In 1st year	In 10 years	In 1st year	In 10 years
0	0.50	2.05	0.90	2.83
5	0.09	1.46	0.13	1.56
10	0.12	2.33	0.12	4.18
15	0.18	2.92	0.30	7.38
20	0.22	2.96	0.77	7.76
25	0.16	3.57	0.39	6.73
30	0.17	4.53	0.32	7.30
35	0.21	6.05	0.35	9.04
40	0.26	9.84	0.49	13.87
45	0.45	17.03	0.68	21.74
50	0.73	27.55	1.08	33.66
55	1.19	37.76	1.54	53.15
60	1.49	58.02	2.15	81.42
65	2.01	81.21	3.16	123.47
70	3.63	124.34	5.94	190.49
75	6.84	207.69	10.44	318.34
80	10.73	340.79	17.21	506.75
85	24.26	576.71	36.40	736.26
90	76.08	860.22	98.22	908.15

Source: Society of Actuaries, 1990–1995 Select and Ultimate Mortality Table (revised May 2, 2002), available at www.soa.org.

stated in deaths per 1,000 per time interval. It should be noted that life insurance expected death rates are lower than those for the general population for standard underwriting classes because of bias introduced by any selection process.

The table showing the number of expected deaths per year (or any other chosen period of time) moves us toward an understanding of medical underwriting. A habit such as smoking or medical condition is important to medical underwriters because it causes a significant increase in expected mortality. Most diseases, risk factors, and tobacco use increase the death rate in a consistent fashion during each interval. For

Table 4.4
Number of Expected Deaths per 1,000 General Population Men per Year for Nonsmokers and Smokers

Age (yrs)	Nonsmoker	Smoker
30	0.32	0.68
50	1.08	2.16
70	5.94	11.98

example, it was once thought that smoking simply shortened the end of life. However, a seminal study by State Mutual Insurance Company in the 1970s demonstrated that smoking almost doubled the mortality at every age. Smoking a pack of cigarettes per day at least doubles the death rate at any given age (Doll 1994). If we examine the effect of smoking on the number of expected deaths, the resulting annual mortality would look like table 4.4.

The number of expected deaths in a group of 1,000 people is low, particularly for young ages. An insurer would expect one death per 5,000 women age thirty in one year. This explains why an impairment that increases mortality by only one extra death per 1,000 per year is important in this age group.

Insured Mortality Tables

A life insurance company has tables for each risk category sorted by age, gender, rating, and expected duration of the contract. Life expectatancy for people in the best category will be better than that in a general population table because of the impact of risk selection or underwriting. In most companies, over 90% of all applicants are issued insurance at standard rates or better. In most companies, general population mortality numbers approximate the mortality expectation in the second or third best pricing category.

Insurers use expected mortality rates per 1,000 people to determine underwriting ratings and pricing. An impairment that doubles the mortality expectation per year will double the death portion of a life premium. Most impairments, risk factors, or diseases, such as smoking, exert the same mortality pressure at every age.

The second major pricing system is the use of flat extras, or a charge per $1,000 of coverage for a set number of years to cover a defined extra rate of expected deaths. Flat extras are most common for avocations such as parachuting, in which the risk of extra death is present only as long as the applicant participates in that activity. Similarly, some diseases, such as cancer, have a high death rate for a short period after diagnosis and then return to background mortality rate. These conditions may be considered to have a constant number of extra deaths per 1,000.

Company actuaries use these same tables to study the company's actual mortality experience, which gives an assessment of the underwriting and pricing. Every year actuaries determine the number of applicants rated in each group or class and the number of actual deaths the company experienced for each duration. If all of the lives were accurately underwritten, actuaries should find the distribution of deaths equal to the underwriting classification results and pricing objectives. The actuary and claims staff should observe that the number of observed deaths for people of any age is lowest in the preferred class and increases with increased ratings. A result other than this would call for a relook at the underwriting tables, staff, or rating manuals.

Risk Selection and Mortality

Application of insurance mortality tables requires a different understanding of mortality than is common in clinical medicine. Clinical medicine is likely to write "a new treatment given to forty-year-olds produced an excellent result with 95% of patients alive after ten years." This translates to fifty deaths per 1,000 over ten years. If we compare these numbers with an insured standard population, the difference becomes quite marked. As seen in table 4.3, the expected ten-year mortality for forty-year-old women is 9.84 deaths per 1,000. The study population had a mortality rate that was 500% higher than the standard insurance population.

We can continue the example and add crude pricing data to illustrate the magnitude of the effect. Let us assume that we have two groups of 1,000 forty-year-old women, one disease free (group A) and one with disease that has 95% ten-year survival (group B). All individuals want to purchase $100,000 of ten-year term life insurance that costs $125 per year. The insurer will pay $100,000 to the survivors of anyone who dies within the ten-year period even if that death occurs the day after the policy was issued.

In this simple example, individuals in group B should each pay $500 annually (or four times the standard rate) for their insurance because that is the cost of their total death benefits paid. Alternatively, if everyone is grouped together, as would occur in a nonunderwritten guaranteed issue population, the average cost of insurance would be $300 to cover the death benefit alone. However, if insurance costs $300 per $100,000 of coverage, some women in group A will consider the cost too high and not buy the coverage. This creates a cost spiral.

Health and Disease to a Medical Underwriter

An underwriter has only one opportunity to rate the applicant and this rating applies for the duration of the contract. An underwriter may be asked to reconsider and reduce a rating if the applicant's health has improved or the disease treated; however, an underwriter cannot increase the rating regardless of what happens to the applicant's medical condition.

Most applicants are in good health, and over 90% are insured at standard rates or better. Many applicants have excellent risk profiles and very low expected mortality. Many standard applicants have minor risk factors such as borderline cholesterol or minimally elevated blood pressure, minor genetic mutations, or genetic heterozygosities that are not significant enough to increase expected mortality.

Some applicants have risk factors that predict for development of future disease and are likely to cause significantly increased mortality. Examples of such predictive risk factors are an elevated total cholesterol level of 280 mg/dl with a decreased high-density lipoprotein of 35 mg/dl (atherosclerosis and coronary artery disease), blood pressure of 142/96 mm Hg (stroke and heart failure), and homozygosity for the C282Y genotype in the HFE gene (iron storage disease or hemochromatosis). Each of these examples carries an increased mortality risk without treatment; however, all of them can be treated. Effective treatment lowers expected mortality back to standard rates.

Many applicants have a known disease history. An acute one-time disease such as appendicitis is of no to minimal interest to a medical underwriter. Applicants may have diseases or medical conditions that can be successfully treated, such as familial hypercholesterolemia, one of the most common and best studied genetic diseases known, that can be effectively treated with prescribed cholesterol-lowering agents and lifestyle modifications. Other diseases are chronic and may have increased mortality even with treatment; for example, diabetes mellitus, a chronic treatable condition that has significantly increased mortality and morbidity. Antithrombin III deficiency, the inherited tendency to form venous blood clots spontaneously, carries an increased mortality unless anticoagulants are prescribed.

The smallest group of medical conditions or diseases consists of conditions that so significantly increase mortality that they are not insurable at reasonable rates. They include metastatic malignancy, congestive heart failure, and Duchenne muscular dystrophy. The increased mortality risk makes issuing a life insurance policy at an affordable rate to these individuals extremely unlikely.

The insurability of a disease depends on its clinical course, severity, the patient's compliance with treatment, and response to treatment. For example, not all patients with ulcerative colitis have the same mortality or risk. Their risk of colon cancer is increased, and many of them undergo frequent colonoscopies to assess for dysplasia or malignancy. Some patients have a prophylactic colectomy to eliminate the risk of colon cancer. Others, for inexplicable reasons, do not have follow-up examinations and may not even regularly visit a physician. Each of these three types of patients with ulcerative colitis presents different risks based solely on their medical care and clinical follow-up. The same logic holds for individuals who have inherited the allele for hereditary nonpolyposis colon cancer (HNPCC), a dominantly inherited condition that increases the risk of colon cancer. The risk of cancer in these applicants with a family history meeting the Amsterdam criteria is 50% (dominantly inherited) times the penetrance of disease. These individuals usually know they are at risk because of a family history of early colon cancer. Screening colonoscopies starting at an early age and colectomy if necessary are appropriate treatments that increase insurability. In fact, it was calculated that a screening colonoscopy in patients with known HNPCC will add seven to nine years to life expectancy (Vasen et al. 1998).

Increasingly, underwriters are seeing long-term survivors of treated disease in whom the primary risk is a complication of therapy. Many childhood leukemias can be treated successfully and cured, and insurers are now seeing adult applicants alive and well twenty years after the diagnosis and successful treatment. These adult survivors no longer have the risk of the primary tumor; however, they may carry a risk of developing a second cancer depending on the toxicities of treatment.

The Underwriting Process

Underwriters assess the entire medical history, noting significant medical factors that are both positive and negative. They determine the total net rating by adding debits and credits for each risk factor or impairment. In many, but not all, companies a debit is equal to 1% increase in mortality. A credit reflects a favorable risk factor.

Underwriters use tables based on actuarial studies to determine the expected mortality of a risk factor or impairment. The Society of Actuaries has done several large intercompany mortality studies on impairments such as build, blood pressure, and liver enzymes. In addition, the clinical literature contains many good longitudinal studies of mortality that lend themselves to actuarial analysis.

The excess death rate for various diseases or risk factors can be determined from industry, actuarial, or large clinical studies. Clinical studies have determined the mortality of many diseases. For example, the mortality of most cancers is captured in large national databases such as the Surveillance, Epidemiology, and End Results program of the National Cancer Institute, the most authoritative source of information on cancer incidence and survival in the United States. Published insurance studies reviewed data from pooled intercompany mortality figures. One example is the intercompany study of alcohol and liver enzymes (Titcombe et al. 2001). Some large insurers also do their own mortality studies of impairments.

Companies analyze data actuarially to determine total mortality or excess death rate sorted by age and gender. Total mortality is the

Table 4.5
Comparative Life Insurer Rating Table

	Debit (% extra mortality)	Total mortality (%)	Final table rating
55-year-old man with no adverse (ratable) risk factors and standard population	0	100	Standard
Obesity (BMI 35)	100	200	B
Crohn disease, controlled with drugs	100	200	B
50% lesion seen on coronary angiogram	100	200	B

Notes: BMI, body mass index; B, second rating classification.

standard mortality plus additional mortality for the adverse risk factor, medical condition, or disease. Determining extra mortality associated with some common cancers or heart disease is relatively straightforward. Some impairments are so uncommon that actuarial data are not available, but statistical data on survival are known or can be surmised from approximate or similar disease states and known complications of the impairment. Rare disorders include diseases such as fascioscapulo-humeral dystrophy and the six subtypes of Ehlers-Danlos syndrome. These are compared with known mortality benchmarks and their clinical progress is assessed for each applicant. Applicants with known disease can and do obtain life insurance at a rate appropriate for their risk. Companies may differ in their assessment of risk, so it is worth while to apply to several to obtain the best possible offer.

Of interest, many risk factors and diseases have similar effect on the expectation of death. Companies do not attempt to classify and rate different groups within each disease or impairment. Rather, they classify applicants with different disorders into groups with similar expected rates of mortality. For example, a fifty-five-year-old applicant with stable Crohn's disease has about the same mortality as a fifty-five-year-old with stable luminal irregularities on coronary angiogram (table 4.5).

Medical underwriters have two primary responsibilities: to put business on the insurer's books and to assess the risk accurately. They seek enough information to understand the clinical course of the disease of each applicant. Underwriters must identify applicants with mild, moderate, or severe disease and which individuals responded favorably to treatment or medically recommended follow-up. Properly underwritten business of all rating classes is profitable for the insurer.

Medical Underwriting Requirements

Most differences in mortality expectation for a given age, gender, and smoking status are related to health factors. Risk factors that affect mortality risk are avocation, occupation, and habits such as driving records. Underwriters are interested in understanding the applicant's health status only to establish risk and pricing categories necessary to support the product.

Companies would not underwrite applicants unless it was absolutely essential to the financial structure and viability of the product. Underwriting costs money and takes time. It requires knowledge, expertise, and information. Information about the applicant must be based on a standard database for all applicants, and the applicant must not be allowed to withhold relevant information.

Two underwriting requirements are age and amount of insurance, and discretionary factors. Age and amount requirements are obtained on all applicants of a given age and applying for more than a given amount of insurance. Discretionary requirements are obtained to clarify or further develop a medical history or test finding. Limits triggering either requirement differ from one company to another.

The risk to a company increases in proportion to the amount of insurance and to the increasing age of applicants. In general, the greater the face amount of the policy (death benefit) the greater the need for information to assess the risk. The older the applicant, the higher the expected death rate and the greater likelihood of a significant medical history or abnormal test. Medical underwriters obtain different types of medical information in proportion to the amount of risk they accept.

Insurers are always interested in the applicant's current health condition and significant medical history. Virtually all applications ask questions about current and prior health status including major illnesses or surgeries, current drug therapy, and family history. As the amount of insurance and age increase, insurers are likely to ask for saliva or urine tests to screen for HIV antibody, nicotine metabolites, and drugs of abuse. At even higher amounts, an insurer may also request a blood test to screen for disorders of lipids, glucose, liver, and kidney function, together with weight and blood pressure. At still higher ages or amounts of insurance, insurers may ask for an electrocardiogram, chest radiograph, treadmill electrocardiogram, or statement from the applicant's personal physician.

The discretionary requirement is ordered to clarify a medical history or test result. A medical underwriter may ask for it to help understand a medical condition regardless of the applicant's age or amount of insurance at risk. Usually the purpose is to obtain information to increase certainty and, in many instances, to place the applicant in a more favorable risk classification. Discretionary requirements might include copies of medical records to investigate an important medical history, and additional blood tests or physical examinations.

All medical information that is statistically significant in determining the applicant's health and longevity is important in the classification of risk. Underwriters may identify an increase mortality risk, but many times more medical information provides a better understanding of the medical history and allows them to offer a lower premium.

The Impact of Medical Advances

Over the past fifty years, significant advances in identification of risk factors for future disease, medical care, and treatments led to major improvements in both survival of treated patients and increased life expectancy for the population as a whole. The insurance-buying public has benefited from these advances through cheaper and more widely available life insurance. Insurers incorporated these medical advances by expanding and refining their rating classifications. More Americans are able to obtain life insurance now at more favorable rates today than ever before.

For example, every decade of the last sixty years has brought greater understanding of the causes of coronary artery disease, new testing technologies, new treatments, and decreases in coronary artery death rates. In the middle of the last century, patients with a heart attack were given oxygen and support. In the 1960s coronary care units were first established for centralized and coordinated medical care of these patients, but care was primarily supportive. Electrocardiograms and cardiac exercise stress tests were identified as means to identify and stratify people at risk for a future heart attack. In the 1960s and 1970s, epidemiologists began to understand risk factors for development of future coronary artery disease. Cardiologists began to study coronary anatomy to identify coronary artery obstructions that were amenable to surgery and, later, balloon angioplasty and stenting. The result is that patients with heart disease receive substantially better treatment and have better survival than at any time in the past.

Identifying predictive risk factors and determining treatment to prevent future disease are important parts of standard medical care. Major risk factors are age, gender, cholesterol (particularly elevated low-density and low high-density lipoproteins), smoking, and diabetes. Asymptomatic patients are routinely tested for risk factors for development of heart disease. Some predictive risk factors for coronary artery disease such as hypercholesterolemia are both genetic and environmentally controlled. It is not worth while to separate the underlying cause (genetic or environmental) as long as effective treatments can be given. Both the clinical and insurance underwriting communities are interested in identifying these significant risk factors because they increase the risk of future disease and premature death unless they are treated.

Ordering Medical Tests for Underwriting

Medical underwriters routinely order blood and urine tests according to applicants' age and coverage requirements. On rare occasions and in response to a specific issue, they may request nonroutine or discretionary tests to clarify a medical question. They consider several criteria before requiring either routine or special tests:

• Does the test accurately identify impairment with significant mortality or morbidity implications?
• What is the cost:benefit ratio of the test?
• Is the test understood and accepted by the clinical community?
• Can the test be easily, accurately, reproducibly, and economically performed in large numbers by the laboratory?

• Does the disorder being tested for occur frequently enough in the insurance-buying population to justify the expense of population screening?
• Does the test improve the equity of underwriting by accurately assigning individuals to appropriate risk categories?
• Does the test enhance the value to consumers by keeping insurance costs low and product availability high for most insurance-buying applicants? (adopted from Daniel and Kita 1998, pp. 233–248)

All blood, urine, or saliva tests are obtained with the signed consent of the proposed insured. Virtually all blood samples are tested in one of four large national laboratories specializing in insurance testing. The laboratories are specifically designed with advanced bar code and computer technology and very high-quality control to handle large numbers of specimens. Specimen containers are bar coded at that time of the original blood draw to minimize errors and enable repeat testing. The laboratories keep all blood frozen for thirty days after testing to permit repeat or reflex testing if necessary. The specimens are then destroyed. It has been estimated that over 7 million samples are tested for insurance annually in the United States alone.

Insurance companies demand accurate test results. Large insurance laboratories meet or exceed all federal and state guidelines and are certified by the College of American Pathologists proficiency testing and the Clinical Laboratory Improvements Act (CLIA). In addition, the laboratories routinely repeat abnormal tests on a different machine to verify the results.

Insurance companies are interested in tests that are significant to longevity, and are not looking for spurious reasons to rate applicants. The industry's commitment to high quality and accurate testing protocols, sensitivity to the notification process, and maintenance of confidentiality indicates its understanding of and commitment to quality testing programs.

The Predictive Value of Tests

Insurers understand that, with few exceptions, diseases are not defined by test results. Most abnormal results indicate only a likelihood of a disease. Screening requires understanding the test's sensitivity and specificity, its validity to identify the disease, and its predictive value. The analogy for a genetic test would be identification of a gene and its penetrance.

Genetic (DNA-based) tests may be predictive or diagnostic. A predictive test is analogous to traditional screening tests in that it predicts only an increased risk, but not a certainty, for the development of future disease. It provides information that, if significant, can be used by the clinical community to begin treatment and by the insurance underwriter to assess risk. Breast cancer (BRCA)-1 and BRCA-2 genetic tests are performed in women with a family history of early and frequent breast or ovarian cancer, as these women are at increased risk of inheriting the genetic mutation simply based on family history. A positive test does not mean that a woman has breast cancer or even that she will absolutely develop the disease; she is only at increased risk. Armed with this information, patient and clinician may decide to proceed with prophylactic measures ranging from vigilant screening to find the cancer at the earliest stage, drug therapy (tamoxifen) to reduce the risk, or prophylactic mastectomy and oophorectomy. The medical underwriter will look at the BRCA test result with the same purpose. If a woman with a BRCA mutation applies for life insurance, what is her increased risk based on the best literature, what steps has she taken to reduce her risk, and is she compliant with treatment?

The next, and possibly, largest use of genetic tests will be for diagnostic purposes. Tests are being developed to determine which patients will respond best to which drugs, to differentiate lymphomas and leukemias, and to diagnose colon cancer by testing stool. Today, most men are tested for elevations in prostate-specific antigen, which indicate the possibility of prostate cancer. At this time, no test is available to tell which prostate cancer will progress and which will stay quiescent; however, researchers are working on their genetic differences. When this information is available, it will enable surgeons to decide whether to operate or watch and wait. Today, medical underwriters treat all prostate cancers the same. Future genetic tests differentiating these tumors will enable them to offer a better rate to men with a favorable genetic profile for the disease.

To the best of my knowledge, no life insurer is performing genetic tests at this time. Medical underwriters frequently see genetic test results in clinical records. Most of these tests have less than complete penetrance and do not always indicate the actual presence of a disease. Furthermore, a positive result gives the person information necessary to take steps to treat or prevent the disease. Finally, some genetic tests have no underwriting significance because they have no mortality implications.

Underwriting Family History

It is well established that many diseases are inherited and can be traced through family histories. Occasionally, a medical underwriter will notice an applicant who indicates that a father, uncle, and brother all died of heart disease in their middle forties. This information by itself may not be sufficient to take adverse action on an application. It will tell the medical underwriter to review other risk factors closely for heart disease to see whether the applicant is ignoring his risky family history, or has taken preventive steps to lower his cholesterol, treat his blood pressure, and maintain a normal weight.

Alternatively, a medical underwriter may note a family history of an autosomal dominant disease with significant mortality implications such as adult polycystic kidney disease. In this instance, the family history alone gives each child a 50% chance of inheriting the mutation and developing the disease, which has a shortened life expectancy because of the risk of renal failure and cerebral aneurysms. The medical underwriter will consider the applicant to have additional mortality until the risk of disease is disproved. A physician is likely to order a test to determine whether the patient actually is at risk because of family history. The medical underwriter will also want that information to make an accurate decision.

Availability of genetic tests for these inherited diseases will put pressure on the clinical community to perform the tests in asymptomatic patients. The results will give clinicians and patients valuable information about risk status. Medical underwriters are already seeing these tests performed in some applicants for life insurance.

Some patients will want to use the information from these test results when developing their financial planning. This may lead to changes in the amount or timing of life insurance purchases. It is essential that medical underwriters have access to genetic tests performed based on family history to assess risks accepted by the company, charge correct premiums, and ensure that other policy owners do not unfairly subsidize these applicants.

Conclusion

Risk selection is the major difference between the free market life insurance risk-based product and government programs. Risk selection requires complete and honest sharing of personal information. In return, the underwriter is responsible for accurately assessing risks consistent with sound actuarial principles or reasonably anticipated experience. The insurer must equitably price products so that each group is self-supporting.

A limitation on the underwriting process upsets the equilibrium of the system. If an applicant withholds information important to risk selection, or is permitted by regulation to withhold important information, the person (or, in the case of life insurance, the estate) will gain an unfair advantage and a very favorable financial return.

An underwriter who violates sound underwriting principles loses in both directions. An underwriter who underprices the real risk (does not recognize a medical risk and accepts it in the standard or better class) will have assumed excess deaths that will show as financial liabilities. An underwriter who overprices risk will lose business to competitors who are more accurate. More than one insurer has suffered financial difficulty because of overly aggressive or incompetent underwriting.

Medical risk selection is the basis of the sound and fair life insurance system in the United States. Advances in medical testing and technology have made insurance more affordable and more widely available to more Americans than ever before. Future developments of genetic testing and genetic medicine should continue this trend toward a healthier America and continued improvements in life insurance availability and affordability for a new generation.

References

Black, K. and Skipper, H. D., Jr., Life Insurance 12th ed. Englewood Cliffs, NJ: Prentice-Hall (1994).

Daniel, P. and Kita, M. W., "Drawing Conclusions From Test Results," in Medical Selection for Life Risks 4th ed., Elder, W. J. and R. D. Brackenridge, eds. Hampshire, UK: Stockton Press (1998).

Doll, R., "Mortality in Relation to Smoking: 40 Years Observations on Male British Physicians," Br. Med. J. 309: 901–911 (1994).

Nowlan, W., "Life Insurance and Genotype Discrimination: An Appeal for Objectivity," Science 297: 195–196 (2002).

Titcombe, C. et al., "Alcohol Abuse and Liver Enzymes: Results of an Intercompany Study of Mortality," J. Insurance Med. 33: 277–289 (2001).

Vasen, H. F. A. et al., "A Cost Effectiveness Analysis of Colorectal Screening for Hereditary Nonpolyposis Colorectal Carcinoma Gene Carriers," Cancer 82: 1632–1637 (1998).

Vital Statistics of the United States, www.cdc.gov/nchs/fastats/lifexpec.htm (2003).

5

Genetic Risks and Mortality Rates

J. Alexander Lowden

The Human Genome Project (HGP) has had a tremendous impact on our understanding of basic human biology. By uncovering the specific genes associated with hundreds of diseases, it changed the way we look at the future health risks of individuals and is beginning to point to ways to mitigate those risks. Future health risks are a major concern for life insurance underwriters who presently attempt to determine life expectancy of applicants based on experience. The possibility that insurers might use genetic testing in risk assessment raises concerns in several quarters. Many of these concerns are based on misunderstandings about the insurance underwriting process.

I hope to dispel some of those fears by showing that some common inherited conditions can be underwritten and that individuals carrying specific mutations can be insured at reasonable cost. I do not address issues of the right of the insurer to access test information or the need to test applicants, but assume that the insurer requires the same knowledge of inherent risks borne by the applicant as the applicant has.

Why Would Life Insurers Consider Genetic Testing?

Before offering coverage to an applicant, life insurers attempt to identify factors that may shorten the person's usual life expectancy at a given age. If identifiable risks exist, the underwriter uses actuarial and medical information to calculate life expectancy and determine an appropriate premium. Genetic tests may offer a means to identify future health risks (Collins 1999) and potentially could improve those calculations. At the present time most genetic tests for predisposition to disease lack valid actuarial information. The likelihood of developing a disease when a mutation in a particular gene is identified is often uncertain. More important, the risk may be greatly altered in the future as we learn how to use genetic knowledge to lower it.

There are many different types of life insurance products and their particular features play different roles in determining the price of each one. Whereas most of the cost of insurance can be determined from experience, actuarial tables, and corporate business practices, expected survival varies with the state of health of the applicant and consideration of future health risks. Because life expectancy is defined as the age at which half the insureds will have died, it is a moving target that increases with the age of the individual at the time of application. To estimate an individual's life expectancy, underwriters consider medical history, current health status, laboratory test results, family history, and lifestyle.

Risk is increased in applicants who have not experienced a clinical event, such as myocardial infarction, but who have evidence of risk in their medical status. Obesity and untreated hypertension trigger an added premium because they are associated with early mortality. Some laboratory tests may also indicate increased risk. Elevated cholesterol, indication of hepatitis C infection, or early evidence of diabetes can be uncovered in people who are otherwise in apparent good health but who, on the basis of a laboratory test showing such a disorder, can be expected to have a shortened life expectancy. Their insurance premiums must reflect the added risk.

The primary goal of medical underwriting is therefore to anticipate the impact of health history and current health status, including laboratory tests, on survival. Unanticipated events do occur. That is one of the reasons for purchasing insurance, but underwriters try to determine what is likely to happen to an applicant and price a policy accordingly. Genetic testing brings a somewhat different aspect to this picture. It potentially provides information about risks that are not anticipated and that may be unrelated to medical or family history.

Causes of death vary with age. Accidental death or trauma is a major factor in younger people, heart disease in middle and later life, and cancer in older people. Almost all mortality, however, has a genetic basis

Table 5.1
The Genetic Basis of Mortality

Genetic basis	Number of deaths/100,000 lives
Chromosomal	380
Single gene defects	2,000
Somatic mutations	24,000
Multifactorial disease	64,600

Source: Kaback (1998).
Notes: Most mortality in early infancy is the result of genetic defects. Later in childhood and early adult life, trauma and infections play a greater role.

(table 5.1). Our knowledge about how mutations are linked to disease has escalated in a logarithmic fashion in the past few years. The HGP will provide many new insights into mechanisms of disease and will continue to identify genes associated with early mortality.

Some genetic tests could possibly bring changes to underwriting decisions. In a person with no family history and no medical history, a series of tests might be able to predict an increased risk of unanticipated disease (Collins 1999). Will, or should, insurers have the right to this information? How will they use it if they do acquire it? To approach the answers to these questions, let us consider knowledge of some common genetic diseases that may lead to early mortality in adults. People with many of these disorders can be underwritten and, for the most part, offered insurance at affordable rates. The secret to what might appear speculative underwriting practice is in knowing the risk and doing something to mitigate possible loss.

Making lifestyle changes or therapeutic decisions may not alter one's genetic risk today, but we live in a world in which scientific discoveries occur at an ever-increasing rate. If an individual has a fatal genetic mutation today, will new developments lead to new methods of management or treatment in the next ten years? Will the mutation have been expressed before new therapy is available? The HGP was not devised to bring new genetic tests to market, but to use genetic information to improve health. In time, people who have genetic tests and know they have certain health risks will be better off than their untested peers for, with knowledge, will come the ability to prevent mutant gene expression.

Thus, predicting future scientific developments as well as health risks based on new information makes medical underwriting extremely difficult.

Protective Value

When insurers spend money to investigate the insurability of an applicant, they try to determine the protective value of the expense. Is the information worth the cost of testing? A typical application form asks questions about the applicant's health and financial status. Application forms cost money to design, register, and produce. They must be completed by brokers, agents, or teleunderwriters, all implying a cost to the insurer. The forms are cost effective, however, because they provide valuable information about the risk and help the underwriter determine how to rate the policy.

Testing has its own costs—of collecting specimens, conducting the test, interpreting results, and relating that interpretation to a relative risk. To justify these costs, actuaries calculate their protective value (Bergstrom 1998). They consider the face amount at risk, anticipated life expectancy of the insured, cost of selling the policy and underwriting the risk, possibility that the policy may lapse before claim, cost of maintaining the policy in force, cost of reserves, accumulated value of the invested premium, and other factors particular to the policy type. It is not a simple exercise.

Test methodology changes almost daily, and cost considerations today may be meaningless tomorrow, but at the present time the average total cost of all laboratory tests for an insurance applicant, including sample collection, is well under $100. Insurers could not sustain a doubling of that cost without increasing premiums. The cost of a molecular genetic test (examining DNA fragments to identify mutations in specific genes) still lies in the hundreds, if not a few thousand dollars (table 5.2). New technologies will examine oligonucleotide fragments and identify point mutations, and do so for many different mutations at the same time. Technology is driving our ability to test for mutations faster than we can expand our ability to comprehend the interplay of several genes and environmental factors that may cause specific diseases. The costs for

Table 5.2
The Cost of Genetic Tests, 2002

Test	Disease	Laboratory	Cost/test ($)
BRACAnalysis	Breast, ovarian cancer	Myriad Genetics	2,580
Colaris	Colon cancer	Myriad Genetics	1,950
CardiaRisk	Cardiovascular	Myriad Genetics	295
Melaris	Melanoma	Myriad Genetics	795
HFE	Hemochromatosis	Kimball Genetics	125
APO E	Alzheimer	Athena Diagnostics	279
SOD-1	Familial ALS	Athena Diagnostics	595
Huntington	Huntington	Athena Diagnostics	325

Note: ALS, amyotrophic lateral selerosis.

these new technologies are falling, and it is reasonable to expect that in a very few years the cost of a battery of genetic tests will be similar to that of a battery of clinical chemistry tests today.

Part of the calculation of protective value is the cost of the test and part, its interpretation. When mutations are rare, fewer tests will be performed and the cost per test for reagents is likely to be high. Furthermore, because the mutation is rare, experience with the test results will be limited and interpretation may be uncertain. To provide protective value, however, tests must not only be inexpensive but the results must be meaningful. It will take time to understand the significance of a group of interacting mutations, the role of environmental influences on those mutations, and the resultant penetrance of the combination. New test formats are intriguing but they do not offer much value to insurance underwriters at this time. In a generation, they clearly will.

Determining the protective value of a genetic test is relatively difficult. First, the number of tests that have a significant impact on human mortality is limited. Second, penetrance of most mutations is variable because we do not understand all the contributing factors. Most important, however, we do not know how the effect of most mutations can be mitigated by lifestyle change or other preventive measures or treatments. Calculating the protective value of doing the tests can therefore become onerous and the determination may be open to considerable question. To calculate protective value, one must have some expected concept of outcome. Unfortunately, with rare genetic mutations, outcomes for unaffected individuals are often uncertain.

Genetic Review

It is not my intention to write a treatise on current understanding of the transmission of genetic risks, as the literature is replete with such articles (Kaback 1998; McKusick 2001; Rosenthal 1994; Schwartz 1994). A few salient points must be understood, however, in order to develop concepts of how an underwriter could fairly and effectively use genetic data.

Much has been written about definitions of genetic testing (Lowden 1999). The HGP initiated a flood of new test protocols (Mir and Southern 2000; Traverso et al. 2002) that completely revolutionized the way we contemplate variations in the genome. It is thus practical to think of a genetic test as a measure of change from the wild-type or common form of inherited information. The test may measure a change in nucleotide sequence or a change in the physical phenotype of an individual as well as many other parameters between these extremes. Changes that affect the nucleotide sequence may be inherited from a parent (germline mutations) or they may develop in a few cells or an organ in postnatal life (somatic mutations). Some tests of change in nucleotide sequence are better performed by examining the product of the gene. For example, measuring enzyme activity is the simplest way to diagnose many inherited diseases of childhood (Scriver et al. 2001), but new assays of truncated expressed protein may be much more informative in somatic mutations where the specimen contains mixtures of mutant and wild-type cells (Traverso et al. 2002).

The paradigm for discussions of the effect of genetic testing on insurance applicants has usually been to select an extremely rare single gene defect that has no known treatment and use the model to devise strategies to cover all forms of genetic disease. Huntington disease is a typical example. Symptoms develop in otherwise healthy adults, progress slowly, and are irreversible. Death occurs in about the sixth decade and cannot be prevented. Because of early mortality, the at-risk person appears uninsurable except at very high rates. There is a litany of reasons not to test this individual: the person may not want to know about the risk, is being discriminated against for something beyond his or her control, or is currently well. In practice, people at risk for Huntington disease are rarely reviewed by underwriters. The incidence of the disease is about 1:10,000 individuals in North America. In spite of its rarity, some individuals are at risk for Huntington disease. Should they receive special consideration in underwriting? Is it fair to inquire about their private family information? Is it fair to consider the risk of disease that has not yet expressed itself? Is it fair to ask others to pay the added cost of insuring someone with a high risk of early death?

Whereas most mortality arises from genetic disease (see table 5.1), only a small fraction results from single-gene mutations and these usually arise in early childhood. The rare untreatable neurologic conditions that occur in adult life provide scope for heated bioethical discussion, but in insurance terms they are so infrequent that they usually never come to the attention of an underwriter. Single-gene diseases are rare and should not be used as the model on which to base legislation about all genetic testing.

To consider strategies for managing genetic risk in insurance underwriting it is essential that concepts of multifactorial disease and somatic mutations be clearly understood. Although single-gene disorders are rare, diagnostic tests for them are easy to develop and understand. Only one gene, or one gene product, has to be assayed. Because a gene may have mutations at many different sites in different people, the test may involve looking at several nucleotide sequences from the same gene. Usually only a few pathologic mutations predominate. Cystic fibrosis has hundreds of mutations, but only a handful are found with any frequency. Screening tests for prospective parents usually only include about twenty-five to thirty mutations. Specific mutations for most genes are usually found in family, racial, or geographic isolates. For example, the breast cancer (BRCA) 1 gene has over 200 known mutations, but 3 predominate in Ashkenazi Jews.

Mutations

Mutations are changes in the sequence of nucleotides in the DNA strand. They may occur in the expressed portion or exon of the gene or in intervening sequences or introns that lie between exons. Mutations in the exon may lead to changes in the sequence of amino acids in the gene product or peptide chain, whereas those in the intron may interfere with transcription of the genetic message. These nucleotide changes may be inherited from a parent or may develop when nucleotides are altered after conception. Inherited or germline mutations are found in all cells of the body, but the postconception or somatic changes are usually confined to specific cells, tissues, or organs. Genetic tests for germline mutations can thus be performed on any cellular source: white blood cells, buccal scrapings, skin cells, or biopsy tissues from organs at risk. Somatic mutations must be identified in the organ in which they arise. Thus, whereas inherited mutations in the BRCA1 gene may give rise to breast cancer, they can be identified in any cellular source. Most breast cancer, on the other hand, is the result of genetic changes that are largely confined to the breast and will not be detected by studying white blood cells.

Germline Mutations   An individual acquires half his or her genome from one parent and half from the other. The genome contains many mutations. Most are single nucleotide polymorphisms (SNPs), in which one nucleotide is replaced by another. This simple change may have no pathological effect. For the RNA codon UGU, a change of the last nucleotide to UGC will not change the amino acid (cysteine) in the resultant protein. If, however, the final nucleotide is G (UGG) the triplet codes for a different amino acid, tryptophan. Substitution of a neutral ring structure for the sulfhydryl group of cysteine may greatly alter the tertiary structure of the protein and thus its function.

In sickle cell disease a mutation in position 6 in the globin protein in hemoglobin A_1 (GAA to GUA) changes the amino acid from glutamic acid to valine (the molecular biologist uses a code, G6V, to indicate the change of the amino acid in position 6) forming a different hemoglobin (HbS) in which the nonpolar valine forms hydrophobic interactions with other HbS molecules to polymerize at low oxygen concentrations. This simple SNP has profound implications for the affected individual. These mutations are called missense mutations.

Single base pair changes may also produce codons that do not have an amino acid counterpart. UGA, UAA, and UAG are called stop codons because when present, they halt the process of transcription. When these triplets appear because of substitution in the nucleotide sequence of an exon they are termed nonsense mutations. The protein from a gene with a stop codon is shortened or truncated.

When a nucleotide is deleted from the sequence, nucleotides after the deletion have an altered coding sequence. Amino acids determined by the altered coding change and produce a resultant peptide with a different structure, usually a protein without the function of the normal or wild type. Single nucleotide deletions are the cause of frameshift mutations.

Many genes have repeating copies of the same sequence. This sequence repeat structure is called a microsatelite and it produces a string of repeats of the same amino acid (or amino acids, depending on the number of nucleotides in the repeated sequence) in the resultant protein. In Huntington disease the triple-repeat CAG is expanded from the usual 6 to 35 repetitions to sequences that may be repeated as often as 100 times. CAG is the code for glutamine but the reason why a longer string of glutamines affects the Huntington protein is not clear. Several neurological diseases result from triplet expansion mutations. They are transmitted as autosomal dominants in which the mutation is present on only one chromosome.

Somatic Mutations   Not all disease is caused by simple changes in the primary DNA sequence. Epigenetic changes may also play a role (Ponder 2001). Hypermethylation of some residues may lead to loss of function of a gene. The normal breakdown and repair of genes may become disrupted, leading to loss of transcription. Methylation frequently occurs in CpG islands (doublets of cytosine-guanine) in promoter regions in somatic cells. This change silences some genes such as VHL, p16, and perhaps BRCA1.

DNA is subjected to many damaging insults and as a result a complex repair mechanism is essential to conserve the sequence integrity. Oxidative damage may convert a C to a U. Depurination may remove the base from a nucleotide while leaving the sugar-phosphate backbone intact. Methylation, particularly of guanosine, produces a highly carcinogenic change in DNA. Ultraviolet light may lead to cross-linking of pyrimidimes along one strand of the DNA. In most instances these mutations can be excised and repaired by the body, but in some they persist. Resultant mutations may lead to disease. A special group of repair genes is responsible for correcting the errors, and individuals who have mutations in repair genes may take many years to display overt pathology. Xeroderma pigmentosa is an example. These patients are photosensitive and highly susceptible to skin cancers. Defects in one of a series of eight different DNA repair genes may be responsible for this disorder.

During the replication process in cell division, occasional mistakes are made in the sequence. A series of enzymes is responsible for identifying these mismatches, excising the nucleotide(s), and replacing them with others in correct sequence. Mismatch repair genes may have mutations and become unable to carry out their function. Hereditary nonpolyposis colon cancer (HNPCC) results from an autosomal dominant mutation in one of at least three mismatch repair genes (MLH1, MSH2, and PMS2). The individual has a germline mutation on only one of a pair of genes. The gene at the same locus on the other chromosome is normal. Disease does not develop until adult life and then only in some individuals who carry the mutation. It is believed that a somatic mutation occurs in the normal allele at some time in life, perhaps related to dietary or other environmental exposure. The phenomenon called loss of heterozygosity is a somatic mutation coupled with a germline mutation to produce a disease. It likely accounts for pathologic changes in many, if not most, so-called autosomal dominant diseases. Because this change is random (or at least not absolute), in many instances all individuals with a dominant mutation do not develop signs of the disease. The frequency with which a specific disease develops is termed penetrance and it is highly variable in different families with the same dominant mutation. Huntington disease is virtually 100% penetrant, but BRCA1-related cancer varies from 35% to 80% in penetrance.

Determining penetrance is difficult. A review of published data on BRCA penetrance shows that different authors assign values ranging from 26% to 74% (Begg 2002). These differences are explained on ascertainment bias. Some studies indicated high levels of penetrance but were done in cohorts tested because they came from high-risk families, with many members having breast or ovarian cancer. Other studies with lower penetrance were done without regard to family history. In considering these differences, it was pointed out that BRCA mutations are not solely responsible for the development of the cancer, and although considered as a single-gene defect, the pathology is actually multifactorial (Begg 2002).

Classic Mendelian rules of genetic transmission have come under scrutiny in recent years. Whereas most single-gene disorders that affect mortality in younger adults are transmitted as autosomal dominant, it is becoming clear that loss of heterozygosity, imprinting, and the effect of other mutations, for example, all play a role in penetrance and expression of these mutations.

SNPs One of the most active areas of genetic research involves the search for SNPs, which are found throughout the genome. One of the earliest SNPs to be described was the G6V mutation in the globin gene of sickle cell disease. A startling observation from the HGP was that the genome has at least 5.3 million SNPs (Patil et al. 2001), 1 occurring every 600 base pairs. Most of them do not cause disease or interfere with protein function; they are true polymorphisms that make each of us different. The SNPs in conserved sequences (haplotypes) are present in all chromosomes. Those in mitochondrial DNA and in the Y chromosome have been used extensively by anthropologists to trace human migration. The SNPs may well be used to identify subgroups of people who will or will not respond to certain medications or carry increased risk of dying from a multifactorial disease.

For most genetic disease, transmission is much more complex than that in simple Mendelian single-gene diseases. These disorders result from mutations in more than one gene, with or without effects of the external environment. Transmission is called multifactorial. In those individuals a demonstrated mutation in one or more genes may or may not cause disease. In most multifactorial disease, we know little of the extent of genetic mutations that are responsible and less about the impact of differing mutations on overall penetrance.

Are Genetic Tests Different from Other Laboratory Tests?

Most standard laboratory tests are simple chemical or immunological assays. They cost a few dollars to perform and are sold in a highly competitive market. Reagents for certain specific reflex tests (hepatitis antibodies, prostate-specific antigen) may cost a few dollars but these tests are usually performed in less than 1% of insurance applicants and only in those with specific indications. They are characterized by high predictive value of morbidity and implied mortality risk, and are considered to have excellent protective value by most insurers. Furthermore, standard tests and resultant reflex assays now in use characterize risks that are understood not only by the investigating underwriter but also by the proposed insured. If told that his or her cholesterol is high, the applicant knows the result indicates an increased risk of heart disease and, more important, knows that something can be done to mitigate that risk. Diet, exercise, and cholesterol-lowering drugs are all responses expected by the public, health care professionals, and insurers. They are assumed to have known value.

Genetic testing is quite different. It is much more specific. It identifies a mutation or several mutations in a gene or genes. The site of the mutation and its particular nucleotide differences are exactly known. On the other hand, the sensitivity, in terms of identifying a mortality risk, is much more tenuous. Furthermore the mutation is not unique to the individual but may be represented in many other family members. Nevertheless, a genetic test is a laboratory exercise to identify possible risk. We do not understand the specifics of that risk well but in time we will. Cholesterol elevations do not give absolute assurance of cardiovascular disease. They only tell us that the risk is increased; BRCA mutations are similar. Both test results can be underwritten because underwriting implies probable, not absolute, risk.

When considering genetic mutations, it is common to hear the phrase "but it is not his fault that he carries the ... mutation." Traditionally, life insurers have not been concerned with personal "fault" on the part of applicants. For example, clear actuarial data show that on average, smokers will die earlier than nonsmokers. The underwriter does not increase a premium on the grounds that smoking can be stopped and it is the smoker's fault for continuing to do so despite the evidence. The underwriter uses risk tables to determine that smokers have a life expectancy that is two to five years less than that of nonsmokers. The difference in survival translates into a difference in the cost of insurance. Similarly, a genetic mutation may carry an increased mortality risk and thus engender an increased premium.

Practical Genetics—What Can Underwriters Do with Genetic Test Results?

Hundreds of genetic tests could be considered in this section, including single-gene defects and multifactorial disorders. It is not possible to catalog them all and for the purposes of outlining an approach to their use, it is not necessary. For details and references on any particluar genetic defect, I refer the reader to the Web-based version of the genetics compendium Online Mendelian Inheritance in Man (key word OMIM). This extensive database is constantly updated by recognized experts in the disorders. It lists over 10,000 entries, many with several subheadings, and is easily searched with minimal criteria. The listings include many current references and these are hypertext-linked to PubMed for more detail.

Certain diseases are discussed both to show examples of different types of genetic disease and to outline approaches for assessing the effect of a genetic mutation on morbidity and mortality. It is my contention that genetic testing should be encouraged as a clinical intervention because many genetic disease risks can be mitigated by heightened surveillance, improved therapy, and changes in lifestyle. These actions can help not only the particular individual but also first-degree relatives: the effect of a genetic test should be positive. Testing should be encouraged by insurers as well because it will lead to better outcomes, adding both a social benefit for policy holders and their families, as well as a monetary benefit to the company. For too long geneticists, bioethicists, epidemiologists, and insurers have wrestled with the spectre of genetic testing as a discriminatory invasion of privacy. It is time we began to consider the long-term benefits it can bring to all parties. Everyone has some genetic mutations. Those who know about their own differences will be in a better position to do something about them. By showing that mutations do not mean denial of coverage, insurers will go a long way toward removing the veil of secrecy and intrigue surrounding testing.

Breast Cancer

Mutations in two genes lead to autosomal dominantly transmitted breast cancer. Both BRCA1 and 2 have been extensively studied and found to have hundreds of mutations, some much more common than others (Easton, Ford, and Bishop 1995; Struewing et al. 1997; Welsch and King 2001). Together they account for less than 10% of all breast cancers. A flash point in controversy between insurers and breast cancer advocates a few years ago, these diseases can now be considered in a new light as understanding of the importance of penetrance and management comes into play. Consider the following facts:

• The risk of breast cancer of all types is about 1:9 for all women.

• The mortality rate is about 30% because most breast cancers are not diagnosed before they reach stage 2 or 3 (National Cancer Institute of Canada 2003).

• Thus the overall lifetime risk for all women of dying from breast cancer is 1:33.

With BRCA mutations, penetrance is now believed to be as low as 40% (Struewing et al. 1997).

• If cancer is diagnosed at stage 1, the mortality is only 10% (National Cancer Institute of Canada 2003). Women who know they carry the mutation could be expected to adopt increased surveillance practices leading to earlier diagnosis. Furthermore, preventive mastectomy and/or treatment with tamoxifen or other chemotherapy will further lower that risk (Eeles et al. 1996).

• Their mortality risk may be on the order of 1:25.

New tests for ovarian cancer may also lower the risk of mortality from that associated tumor (Petricoin et al. 2002). From an underwriting perspective, even in the absence of prophylactic surgery (Eeles et al. 1996) or preventive chemotherapy, the calculated risk for a woman with a BRCA mutation is not much different from the breast cancer risk for all women. The important feature is that a positive test must be associated with a positive management approach: women who know they carry a BRCA mutation can do something about it, those who do not know may have stage 2 or 3 disease before they are diagnosed. Genetic testing for this risk should be encouraged in families with a history of breast or ovarian cancer.

Colon Cancer

Colon cancers arising from HNPCC (OMIM 2002b) and familial APC (OMIM 2002a) mutations are additional examples for which knowledge of the mutation should trigger preventive action. Although these mutations also represent only a small fraction of the total colon cancer burden, the tumors are usually slow growing and can be identified early by colonoscopy in individuals who know they carry a mutant gene. When lesions are identified, the person may be treated with total colectomy and will no longer be at risk. Because of the relatively high frequency of colon cancer (about 14% of all cancer deaths in North America) the cohort of people who know they carry a mutant gene is actually at lower risk than the population at large, provided they undergo regular colonoscopies.

A new genetic test for colon cancer has recently been described (Traverso et al. 2002). Targeting both those who do not carry an inherited mutant gene as well as the group described above, the test searches in stool samples for acquired mutations in the APC gene that are found in all colon tumors. These mutations occur only in about 1 in 250 copies of the APC gene that are shed into the bowel from the tumor. They are not in all cells because these are acquired or somatic mutations. The test dilutes APC gene copies so the mutated forms stand out. This approach may one day supplant occult blood tests that are in use today. The predictive value of the APC test appears much higher than that of occult blood, and it is an excellent example of the use of molecular technology that should be encouraged and supported by both geneticists and insurers.

Diabetes Mellitus

Diabetes mellitus type 2 (DM 2) provides a different approach to the use of genetic information. It is not transmitted as a simple single gene defect but it is clearly genetically determined and probably has a multifactorial etiology. Racial differences are one indication of the genetic basis. Pima Indians in the United States southwest have a 40% lifetime risk of developing DM 2, but the prevalence in white Americans is only about 10% to 15%. Monozygotic twins are reported to have 80% to 100% concordance, whereas the risk in nontwin sibs is 38% and in offspring 33%. The disease arises from insulin resistance and defects in the insulin receptor gene, the insulin receptor substrate, glucokinase, and amylin. These mutations are present in varying prevalences in different population groups, indicating that DM 2 is not one but many diseases with quite different etiologies (Chuang et al. 1998; O'Rahilly et al. 1992; Sakagashira et al. 1996). The mutation alone does not cause the disease, but at least two mutations in association with some environmental factor would appear to be the cause. Will this confusing picture ever lead to useful underwriting information? Perhaps some calculations will identify certain subsets of the DM 2 symptom complex that will have predictive value.

Today, individuals with DM 2 can be well managed with various combinations of diet, exercise, oral agents to increase insulin production or use, injected insulin, angiotensin-converting enzyme inhibitiors, and statins. Although their life expectancy may be slightly curtailed, it is far better than it was in earlier times (Sacco 2002), but the risk must be acknowledged for fair underwriting. The important issue in DM 2 is diagnosis and enrollment into a proper therapeutic regimen. A diabetic in good control will have normal blood glucose, fructosamine, and hemoglobin A_{1c}, and urine free of glucose or microalbumin. If molecular testing becomes the first line of diagnosis at some time in the future, legislation that prevents an insurer from learning results of those tests may preclude knowledge of the risk.

Type 2 DM is one of the most common diseases in adults. If, before the onset of hyperglycemia and symptoms, genetic testing could be done to provide an early warning of risk, it could lead to lifestyle changes that might delay or certainly lessen the morbidity and mortality associated with this syndrome.

Hemochromatosis

Hereditary hemochromatosis is an autosomal recessive disease of iron metabolism. It develops from a mutation in the HFE gene (6p21.3). Two mutations in HFE account for most patients: C282Y, in which cysteine at position 282 in the amino acid sequence is replaced with tyrosine, was the first mutation described; and the second, in which 63 histidine is replaced by aspartic acid (H63D) (Melis et al. 2002). A mutation in a second gene was implicated in some forms of the disease. The transferrin receptor gene 2 (7q22) TfR2 has a nonsense mutation that also leads to an iron overload syndrome (Camaschella et al. 2000).

Hemochromatosis is easily managed with regular phlebotomies to keep iron levels low and prevent secondary complications of iron overload (cirrhosis, diabetes, and adrenal failure). These problems respond poorly to treatment after they have commenced. To achieve optimal management, the diagnosis must be made before onset of symptoms. Several attempts have been made to develop screening programs to identify the individuals with iron overload but they have not been successful. Whereas about 1:200 North Americans have a homozygous HFE mutation, penetrance of the disease is relatively low. Many with mutations will not develop signs of the disease. Individuals with these mutations should be underwritten as standard risks if they have not developed pathological complications. They should be encouraged to participate in a regular blood donor program to mitigate their risk. If they remain untested, the first indication of that risk may be a secondary complication. Hemochromatosis is clearly a disease that warrants screening in early adult life. Again knowledge prevents disease, protecting both the insured and the insurer.

Alzheimer Disease

One of the most common disorders of aging is Alzheimer disease (AD). Estimates indicate that as many as 30% of adults who survive to age 85 will develop signs of the disease. It is more common in women than in men, and in those with lower intelligence and lower education. It occurs less frequently in those who maintain an active as opposed to inactive intellectual lifestyle (Wilson et al. 2002). The relationship of these facts to a genetic basis for the disease seems small. Nevertheless, clear indications of genetic influence exist and thus of predictive testing.

Much has been written about presymptomatic testing for AD risk (Hyman et al. 1996; Roses 1996; Tsuang et al. 1999) based on the observation that apolipoprotein E ε4 (Apo E) alleles are present in high frequency in these patients. The association begs the question of whether this information can be used in a predictive manner. A meeting sponsored by the Alzheimer's Association and the National Institute on Aging in 1995 (reviewed in Roses 1996) made the following conclusions:

• Predictive testing for cognitively intact persons was not recommended.
• APO E genotyping showed promise in the diagnosis of dementia.
• APO E genotyping may be useful in selecting therapies.

These were important conclusions because of considerable confusion in the press and the minds of many interested parties about the role of this assay in risk assessment. Experts at this consensus conference concluded that Apo E ε4 had limited utility as a prognostic indicator for the development of dementia.

Several other genetic mutations have been implicated (St. George-Hyslop 2000) in familial AD (FAD). These include a defect in the gene for β-amyloid precursor protein (21q21), in the presenilin-1 gene (14q24.3), and in the presenilin 2 gene (1q31-q42). All are associated with early-onset, autosomal dominant forms of FAD. Whereas AD occurs rarely in younger adults, these genetic mutations do suggest that preclinical diagnostic testing might be feasible. In reality, only 38% of first-degree relatives develop FAD, indicating incomplete penetrance and thus a role for other genes or environmental factors. The disease does not result from a simple single-gene defect. Performing tests for these genes for risk selection is thus inappropriate because it is bound to identify individuals with mutations who will never develop AD.

At this time, arguments against testing are valid (Skoog 2000), but new forms of treatment may change that. Molecular technologies may provide fancy methods for diagnosing dementia in its early stages, but if the disease is untreatable, it is clearly not fair, at this time, to insist on testing to determine risk of future disease in unaffected people.

Alzheimer disease is a good example of how risk may change with new scientific developments. Many patients who begin to show signs of dementia are treated with cholinesterase inhibitors. The drugs do not arrest the progression of the dementia but they do slow its development. More exciting is work on amyloid-β peptide as a vaccine to reduce the burden of brain amyloid (Janus et al. 2000). This work, carried out in PDAPP transgenic mice, a model of AD, shows great promise and may completely alter the outlook for individuals developing dementia. If it achieves its goals, genetic testing for possible risk of AD may completely change the genetic testing paradigm for this devastating disease. People who can be identified as at risk can be treated before they develop severe dementia.

More imminent, studies in these mice show that injection of a monoclonal antibody against the β-amyloid peptide results in release of β-amyloid into plasma where it can be measured (DeMattos et al. 2002). β-Amyloid begins to accumulate in brains of those who will develop AD at least ten years before demonstrable cognitive deficiency. Will this assay prove to be a good predictive test? It is not a genetic test by most definitions, but by predicting risk in the unaffected well, it would be clearly just as unfair as a DNA test that might indicate this risk.

This example points out one of the problems surrounding legislative attempts to control genetic testing. What is a genetic test? Is measurement of β-amyloid peptide a genetic test? If so, why is measurement of any "standard" analyte (cholesterol, alanine aminotransferase, blood urea nitrogen) any different? All may be elevated in the absence of apparent clinical disease and all predict serious outcomes with various degrees of risk. More important, all, including β-amyloid peptide, may indicate a possible need for treatment to mitigate risk.

Huntington Disease

Much rhetoric surrounding genetic testing and insurance stems from consideration of Huntington disease (HD). It is an autosomal dominant disorder with virtually 100% penetrance. An individual with an affected parent has a 50% chance of developing HD. Early knowledge of the existence of the mutation provides little help as there is no therapy, no way to mitigate the outcome. Because of the inevitability factor many groups think family history of HD should be considered confidential and should not be disclosed to an insurer. The viewpoints are discussed in other chapters, but I propose that, in the absence of testing, applicants at risk for HD can be underwritten in a reasonable manner.

Consider a twenty-five-year-old man whose father developed HD at age thirty-five and died at age fifty. He has a sister with HD onset at age thirty-seven who is alive at age forty-two, and an unaffected brother age thirty-three. He does not want to have a test for HD but does want to buy insurance because he is married and has just purchased a house.

His a priori risk is 50% that he will die by age fifty years. It will be ten to fifteen years until he begins to develop signs of HD, if he carries the mutation. If so, he will have about twenty-five years of life remaining, but if not his life expectancy is another fifty-four years. The average years of life remaining is thus 39.5 years, indicating a mortality of 400% (in actuarial terms the mortality is slightly less because the relationship between dying at 50 and dying at 79 is not a straight line). For this model to work, all at-risk HD offspring must be insured and unaffected ones must maintain their policies in effect even after they know they do not carry the gene. That situation is unlikely.

Insurers can use a different tool to manage this situation. By applying a small, flat, extra rating to the premium for about fifteen years, the 400% mortality risk can be covered. The extra premium in this case would amount to about $2.25 per $1000 of coverage and would be paid by all HD at-risk offspring before those carrying the mutation developed signs of the disease. The risk would be fairly priced. The applicant would be insurable.

This underwriting model can be used for any untreatable disease for which there is a symptom-free period in early adult life. It is fair to the individual with the family history, and it is fair to other insureds who are not asked to carry an extra burden to provide coverage to someone with an unequal risk.

Coronary Artery Disease

Although incredible changes in outcomes have been realized for patients after acute coronary events in the past twenty years, at least half of death claims of most insurers are for heart disease. Typically, the risk is identified on the basis of history, including family history, measurements of serum lipids, and electrophysiological studies, including cardiograms and treadmill stress tests. Total cholesterol, low-density lipoprotein cholesterol (LDL), and high-density lipoprotein cholesterol (HDL) are the mainstays of the investigation from the underwriters' perspective, and indeed, clinical management of serum lipids is the major reason for improvements in outcome (Steinberg and Gatto 1999). Many other tests have been advocated, including high-sensitivity C-reactive protein (Ridker et al. 2000), uric acid (Bickel et al. 2002), Apo B (OMIM 2002c), and the ε2 and ε4 alleles of Apo E (OMIM 2002d), but these have seen little use in insurance underwriting. Despite intensive study and clear indications that myocardial infarctions occur in greater frequency in people with dyslipidemias, at least half of all coronary events develop in individuals with normal lipid levels (Braunwald 1997).

It was suggested that better risk determination would be possible if we understood the genetics of lipid control and endothelial dysfunction. Four major genetic mutations affect serum cholesterol levels (Desjeux 2001) and cause familial hypercholesterolemia:

• A defect in the gene for the LDL receptor protein (LDLR) (Goldstein et al. 1995). Heterozygotes for this mutation are found at a frequency of 1:500 in Caucasians and usually have total cholesterol levels of about 300 mg/dL. Homozygous affecteds are extremely rare (1:1,000,000).
• Familial ligand-defective Apo B 100, another rare defect occurring in 1:1000 or less in most European populations but not at all in Asians and other peoples (Viola et al. 2001).
• ABC transport defects (ABCG5 and ABCG6) are transmitted as recessives, and affected patients accumulate a rare form of LDL that includes sitosterol, a plant sterol, as well as cholesterol (Berge et al. 2000).

• Autosomal recessive hypercholesterolemia in which serum cholesterol levels resemble those in homozgous LDLR, but serum lipids in heterozygous parents are within normal limits (Simons and Ikonen 2000).

There are four genetically different reasons for cholesterol levels to rise, but all are rare. Most high cholesterol levels and most coronary artery disease risk are multifactorial. They probably involve susceptibilty factors that influence lipoprotein uptake or sterol regulation (Desjeux 2001) acting in concert with other genes that may or may not have undergone somatic mutations in adult life. Diet and sedentary lifestyle clearly play a role. Genetic tests to uncover monogenic disorders of cholesterol homeostasis are academically interesting, but for risk assessment, at this time, family history, body mass index, serum lipids, and perhaps high sensitivity c-reactive protein continue to be the best indicators of cardiac risk (Day and Wilson 2001). Management will become more aggressive as the influence of the National Cholesterol Education Program and its Advanced Treatment Program III gain acceptance (Stein 2002). Without knowing specific genes involved, treatment will be similar, if not identical.

Genetics in the Future—Impact on Insurance Practices

The HGP was not developed to design a series of tests for use in predicting life expectancy, but to decrease the morbidity and mortality burden of these sequence errors. Changing medical management of coronary artery disease has had an important effect on life expectancy over the last generation (Steinberg and Gotto 1999). That change will be considered minimal, however, when the new science of pharmacogenomics teaches us how to select correct medication for specific individuals. In like manner, telomerase inhibition may revolutionize our mortality statistics if it can be used to control cancer (Kelland 2000).

If genetic tests are considered only in an unfavorable light, many people will miss the opportunity to modify an impending risk because they think the results will be used unfairly. Genetic test results should be considered in the same way we think about cholesterol assays. They predict dire consequences if the affected person does nothing with the information, but taken as a stepping stone to averting risk, they are valuable. Furthermore when one recognizes that a genetic predictive test has many similarities to nongenetic tests, the confusion arising from attempting to separate genetics into a secret world becomes not only futile but dangerous.

Test results should not just lead to dire predictions about outcome. They should stimulate change. We can expect that information about risk will lead to increasing attempts to protect individuals from their genetic mistakes. Changes in lifestyle, nutrition, and other exposures may decrease risk. Pharmaceutical or surgical management and possibly genetic manipulation may all improve the outcome of those who are aware of their risk.

References

Begg, C. B., "On the Use of Familial Aggregation in Population-based Case Probands for Calculating Penetrance," J. Natl. Cancer Inst. 94: 1221–1226 (2002).

Berge, K. E. et al., "Accumulation of Dietary Cholesterol in Sitosterolemia Caused by Mutations in Adjacent ABC Transporters," Science 290: 1771–1775 (2000).

Bergstrom, R. L., "The Predictive Value of Urine Revisited," On the Risk 14(2): 66–70 (1998).

Bickel, C. et al., "Serum Uric Acid as an Independent Predictor of Mortality in Patients with Angiographically Proven Coronary Artery Disease," Am. J. Cardiol. 89: 12–17 (2002).

Braunwald, E., Shattuck Lecture: "Cardiovascular Medicine at the Turn of the Millennium: Triumphs, Concerns, and Opportunities," N. Engl. J. Med. 337: 1360–1369 (1997).

Camaschella, C. et al., "The Gene TFR2 Is Mutated in a New Type of Haemochromatosis Mapping to 7q22," Nature Genet. 25: 14–15 (2000).

Chuang, L. M. et al., "Role of S20G Mutation of Amylin Gene in Insulin Secretion, Insulin Sensitivity, and Type II Diabetes Mellitus in Taiwanese Patients" [letter], Diabetologia 41: 1250–1251 (1998).

Collins, F. S., Shattuck Lecture: "Medical and Societal Consequences of the Human Genome Project," N. Engl. J. Med. 341: 28 (1999).

Day, I. N. M. and Wilson, D. I., "Genetics and Cardiovascular Risk," Br. Med. J. 323: 1409–1412 (2001).

DeMattos, R. B. et al., "Brain to Plasma Amyloid-β Efflux: A Measure of Brain Amyloid Burden in a Mouse Model of Alzheimer's Disease," Science 295: 2264–2267 (2002).

Desjeux, J. F., "Monogenic Disorders that Cause LDL Cholesterol to Accumulate in Plasma," J. Pediatr. Gastroenterol. Nutr. 33: 119–121 (2001).

Easton, D. F., Ford, D., and Bishop, D., "Breast and Ovarian Cancer Incidence in BRCA1 Mutation Carriers," Am. J. Hum. Genet. 56: 265–271 (1995).

Eeles, R. et al., "Prophylactic Mastectomy for Genetic Predisposition to Breast Cancer: The Proband's Story," Clin. Oncol. 8: 222–225 (1996).

Goldstein, J. L., Hobbs, H. H., and Brown, M. S., "Familial Hypercholesterolemia," in C. R. Scriver et al., eds., The Metabolic and Molecular Basis of Inherited Disease, 7th ed, New York: McGarw-Hill (1995), pp. 1961–2030.

Hyman, B. T. et al., "Epidemiological, Clinical and Neuropathological Study of Apolpoprotein E Genotype in Alzheimer's Disease," Ann. NY Acad. Sci. 802: 1–5 (1996).

Janus, C. et al., "A β Peptide Immunization Reduces Behavioral Impairment and Plaques in a Model of Alzheimer's Disease," Nature 408: 979–982 (2000).

Kaback, M. M., AMA Conference on Genetic Disease, New Orleans, personal communication (1998).

Kelland, L. R., "Telomerase Inhibitors: Targeting the Vulnerable End of Cancer?," Anticancer Drugs 11: 503–513 (2000).

Lowden, J. A., "Ethical Issues Resulting from Genetic Technology," North Am. Actuarial J. 3: 67–82 (1999).

McKusick, V. A., "The Anatomy of the Human Genome. A Neo-Vesalian Basis for Medicine in the 21st Century," JAMA 286: 2289–2295 (2001).

Melis, M. A. et al., "H63D Mutation in the HFE Gene Increases Iron Overload in Beta-Thalassemia Carriers," Haematologia 87: 242–245 (2002).

Mir, K. U. and Southern, E., "Sequence Variation in Genes and Genomic DNA: Methods for Large Scale Analysis," Annu. Rev. Hum. Genet. 1: 329–360 (2000).

National Cancer Institute of Canada, Canadian Cancer Statistics 2003. Toronto: National Cancer Institute of Canada (2003).

Online Mendelian Inheritance in Man, http://www.ncbi.nlm.goc/entrez, "Adenomatous Polyposis of the Colon," APC in OMIM #175100 (2002a).

Online Mendelian Inheritance in Man, http://www.ncbi.nlm.gov/entrez, "Colorectal Cancer, Hereditary Non-Polyposis," HNPCC in OMIM #114500 (2002b).

Online Mendelian Inheritance in Man, http://www.ncbi.nlm.goc/entrez, "Apolipoprotein B," in OMIM #107730 (2002c).

Online Mendelian Inheritance in Man, http://www.ncbi.nlm.goc/entrez, "Apolipoprotein E," in OMIM #107741 (2002d).

O'Rahilly, S. et al., "Insulin Receptor and Insulin-responsive Glucose Transporter (GLUT-4) Mutations and Polymorphisms in a Welsh Type 2 (non-insulin dependent) Diabetic Population. Diabetologia 36: 486–489 (1992).

Patil, N. et al., "Blocks of Limited Haplotype Diversity Revealed by High Resolution Scanning of Human Chromosome 21," Science 294: 1719–1723 (2001).

Petricoin, E. F. et al., "Use of Proteomic Patterns in Serum to Identify Ovarian Cancer," Lancet 359: 572–577 (2002).

Ponder, B. A., "Cancer Genetics," Nature 411: 336–341 (2001).

Ridker, P. M. et al., "C-reactive Protein and Other Markers of Inflammation in the Prediction of Cardiovascular Disease in Women," N. Engl. J. Med. 342: 836–843 (2000).

Rosenthal, N., "Molecular Medicine. DNA and the Genetic Code," N. Engl. J. Med. 331: 39–41 (1994).

Roses, A. D., "Apolipoprotein E and Alzheimer's Disease. A Rapidly Expanding Field with Medical and Epidemiological Consequences," Ann. NY Acad. Sci. 802: 50–57 (1996).

Sacco, R. L., "Reducing the Risk of Stroke in Diabetes: What We Have Learned that Is New?," Diabetes Obes. Metab. 4(Suppl. 1): 27–34 (2002).

Sakagashira, S. et al., "Missense Mutation of Amylin Gene (S20G) in Japanese NIDDM Patients," Diabetes 45: 1279–1281 (1996).

Schwartz, R. S., "A New Series on Molecular Medicine for Clinicians" [editorial], N. Engl. J. Med. 331: 47 (1994).

Scriver, C. R. et al., eds., Metabolic and Molecular Bases of Inherited Disease, 4th ed. New York: McGraw-Hill (2001).

Simons, K. and Ikonen, W., "How Cells Handle Cholesterol," Science 290: 1721–1726 (2000).

Skoog, I., "Detection of Preclinical Alzheimer's Disease," N. Engl. J. Med. 343: 502–503 (2000).

St. George-Hsylop, "Molecular Genetics of Alzheimer's Disease," Biol. Psychiatry 47: 183–199 (2000).

Stein, E. A., "Managing Dyslipidemia in the High-Risk Patient," Am. J. Cardiol. 89(5 Suppl. 1): 50–57 (2002).

Steinberg, D. and Gotto, A. M., Jr., "Preventing Coronary Artery Disease by Lowering Cholesterol Levels: Fifty Years from Bench to Bedside," JAMA 282: 2043–2050 (1999).

Struewing, J. P. et al., "The Risk of Cancer Associated with Specific Mutations of BRCA1 and BRCA2 among Ashkenazi Jews," N. Engl. J. Med. 336: 1401–1408 (1997).

Traverso, G. et al., "Detection of APC Mutations in Fecal DNA from Patients with Colorectal Tumors," N. Engl. J. Med. 246: 311–320 (2002).

Tsuang, D. et al., "The Utility of Apolipoprotein E Genotyping in the Diagnosis of Alzheimer Disease in a Community-based Case Series," Arch. Neurol. 56: 1489–1495 (1999).

Viola, S. et al., "Apolipoprotein B Arg3500Gln Mutation Prevalence in Children with Hypercholesterolemia: A French Multicenter Study," J. Pediatr. Gastroenterol. Nutr. 33: 122–126 (2001).

Welsch, P. L. and King, M.-C., "BRCA1 and BRCA2 and the Genetics of Breast and Ovarian Cancer," Hum. Mol. Genet. 10: 705–713 (2001).

Wilson, R. S. et al., "Participation in Cognitively Stimulating Activities and Risk of Incident Alzheimer Disease," JAMA 287: 742–748 (2002).

6

The Functions of Insurance and the Fairness of Genetic Underwriting[1]

Norman Daniels

One promise of the Human Genome Project is that we will learn much more about the genetic basis of risks to health, normal functioning, and life, thereby reducing the uncertainty we insure ourselves against when we purchase medical, disability, and life insurance. Specifically, scientists may develop screening tests that give us much more accurate information, available from birth or even the time of conception, about our probability of acquiring certain diseases, becoming disabled from a medical condition during our working years, or dying prematurely. Some of this information may be of great value to individuals: it may provide a basis for prevention or early treatment of conditions that would be serious if not addressed, or it may simply reduce uncertainty.

This same information, especially if it is available to individuals, is of value to private insurers in underwriting health, disability, and life insurance. It is in the interest of insurers to evaluate the best information about the risks that people face. How should information that derives from the genome project and related work in molecular biology be used in these different insurance contexts? If insurers find it in their interest to use such information, should they be allowed to do so? Do considerations of fairness or justice militate against the use of genetic information in insurance underwriting? Is genetic information different from other kinds of medical information used in underwriting, or does the fairness of its use stand or fall with the fairness of medical underwriting more generally?

We all know that a rose by any other name is a rose. Is insurance, by any of its names—health, disability, life—still insurance and subject to the same considerations of fairness? It is tempting to think that it is. Private insurers, who are subject to standard economic forces operating in the marketplace for all types of insurance, reinforce this temptation. They remind us about practices we all accept without question and think are reasonable. For example, it seems reasonable for people who face greatest risks of having a car stolen, because they have bought models known to be popular targets of thieves, to pay more for insurance against theft. Similarly, insurers in Massachusetts want to inspect used cars before insuring them; they want to know as much about dents and defects as the owners do before providing coverage against costly repairs. In this case, it seems natural and fair for insurers to be able to find out about prior conditions that insureds know about (it prevents fraud).

From the perspective of insurers, insurance is insurance is insurance, and it is uniformly subject to laws. In this uniform function or risk-management view, individuals have an interest in managing the risks they face, and insurers bring to market instruments through which individuals can purchase the kinds of security they want. These instruments are stable, and a market for them can exist only if insurers have information about risks that is as actuarially sound as possible and is at least as accurate as the information individuals have.

To see the point behind the uniform function view, consider, for example, the risk-management aspect of insurance, ignoring for the moment special moral importance we may attribute to assuring access to health care services. From this perspective, health insurance is only a way for rational economic agents to manage their risks of serious economic losses under conditions of uncertainty. Prudent people buy insurance because they prefer to face modest, predictable losses (premiums) on a regular basis rather than face catastrophic losses at unpredictable times. Absence of information about when losses will occur gives people an interest in pooling risks. When all potential insureds symmetrically lack information, prudent consumers of insurance will have a common interest in sharing their risks.

The situation changes when we acquire information that allows us to disaggregate the risks and sort people into stratified risk pools. For example, suppose we can differentiate the risks covered by homeowners' insurance using information about the construction, age, structural soundness, and location of houses, as well as information about available firefighting facilities and relevant fire safety codes. Or suppose we can differentiate health risks through information about individual medical histories, genetic predisposition to disease or genetic disorders, or behavior, such as smoking. Then, those purchasing insurance will come to see themselves as having distinct rather than common interests. Those whose medical history or behavior leads them to believe that they are at lower than average risk will prefer to pool their risks only with others at comparably low risk, since the lower probability of an adverse event reduces the expected collective pay-out and hence should make it cheaper to buy security. They may not want to subsidize security for those at higher risk. At the same time, those at high risk will seek the bargain in security offered by insurance that pools high- and low risk-individuals. This is called adverse selection.

If they are to remain competitive, insurers must respond to these consumer preferences. They must protect themselves against adverse selection, excluding those at higher risk or charging them higher premiums; then they can aggressively market insurance to those at lower risk who seek security at a lower price. The behavior of insurers thus responds to competitive forces in a particular marketing context, one that assumes insurance—health or otherwise—has the primary function of giving individuals the opportunity to manage risks prudently. This assumption, as we will see, is far from morally neutral. Changing the rules governing marketing, for example, by making medical insurance compulsory and requiring that all premiums be community rated, would not eliminate profit. But justifying those changes requires a different assumption about the function of insurance, for example, that insurance is necessary to guarantee people adequate access to medical care and is not simply an instrument of individual risk management.

The idea that different kinds of insurance may have different social functions, with different implications for the fairness of underwriting practices, we will call the multifunction thesis. It may be reasonable to view fire and theft insurance as simple instruments for risk management. But if, for example, we have strong social obligations to ensure access to anyone who requires medical services, a system of private medical insurance must be integrated into delivery and financing institutions that ensure access to those services. That integration can take place in different ways, but to be effective it may require modifying the rules under which private health insurance is marketed and the types of underwriting permitted.

To decide whether the multifunction thesis is true, we must examine the social function or functions of each type of insurance, consider whether we have social obligations that must be met in carrying out these functions, and determine the implications for modifying the markets accordingly. If we adopt this strategy for thinking about fairness in different insurance markets, saying that insurance is insurance, because private insurance markets for risk-management must obey certain economic laws, appears to beg the question. It begs the question whether we should significantly modify those markets or even replace them with forms of social insurance.

Although the uniform function view has dominated the American insurance scene, even in health insurance, it has come under significant attack. Medical underwriting is widespread in life and disability insurance markets (outside employee group benefit plans). "For the insurer, screening and classification of risks protects solvency by allowing premiums to be set at a level commensurate with those risks. For consumers, underwriting protects the insurer's ability to deliver payment when needed" (American Academy of Actuaries 1998). This medical underwriting has not led to any significant economic or moral objections. The case is dramatically different for health insurance, especially recently, even though medical underwriting is restricted primarily to individual and small group markets, affecting only a minority of those with health insurance. In recent years, the public has come to perceive medical underwriting of health insurance as an important threat to security and fairness. This perception resulted from the expanded use of medical underwriting for individual and small group health insurance during the 1980s, coupled with increasing lack of security about the permanence of employment relations and a growing trend among employers to reduce benefits. Even workers with secure jobs and benefits fear switching jobs, since they may then have difficulty obtaining health insurance because of health risks faced by them or their dependents.

This fear and the resulting employee "job lock" led Congress to enact the Health Insurance Portability and Accountability Act of 1996. The law prohibits employer-based group health plans from charging members different rates or providing different coverage levels based on health status. It also severely limits exclusions based on preexisting conditions. The law does not apply to individual policies, which some suggested should use community rating aimed at prohibiting at least some forms of risk rating.

Opposition to medical underwriting practices rests on both economic and moral considerations. Many have come to believe that excluding people from medical insurance leads to shifting the costs of providing services from the uninsured, who do not pay, to those who are insured (Institute of Medicine 2002). Although most uninsured are not denied coverage because of health risks, those who are so excluded add to the problem of cost shifting, and evidence is growing that the uninsured get too little too late.

Many also think that these exclusions are unfair or unjust. Those who need insurance the most because they face high risks have the hardest time getting it, even though medical care should be distributed according to need (or so most people believe). Even people who are not excluded from coverage but are charged higher than standard rates may face insurmountable economic barriers to access. More generally, risk-rating individual and small group insurance not only erects access barriers for some people, but it embodies the objectionable principle that the sick should bear a disproportionately large burden of the costs of health care. (Copayment requirements of course violate the same principle.) This issue of whether to use community rating is more complicated morally than the issue of risk exclusions: community rating might raise premiums for some young healthy workers, creating access barriers for them if they are low income. More generally, there is also something objectionable about asking poor healthy people to help subsidize the costs of insurance for rich people at higher risk. We return to these complexities in more detail later.

If we are to understand in both theoretical and practical ways what kinds of restrictions these considerations of fairness impose on the use of genetic information for insurance underwriting, we must understand why different types of insurance are perceived in such different ways. We must examine the multifunction thesis systematically. Our strategy here is to consider what arguments from justice or fairness imply that standard underwriting practices for medical insurance are morally objectionable. We will then see if these arguments have reasonable application in the case of disability and life insurance, and thus what fairness requires in the way of policy recommendations in each case.

Before turning to the multifunction thesis, we will address one concept that might be thought to make that thesis irrelevant. According to this concept we are morally obliged to make sure that premiums for insurance of any type reflect the risks of the insured. This obligation applies equally to fire and theft insurance and to health, disability, and life insurance. In effect, this argument from actuarial fairness would imply an obligation to act on the uniform function view that insurance is insurance by any of its names. What is at issue is the permissibility of all medical underwriting. Since medical underwriting based on genetic information is a special case, for most of this discussion we will assume that there is no difference between genetic and other medical information and return to the assumption later.

Actuarial Fairness[2]

Many Americans are denied access to adequate individual or small-group medical insurance, to nongroup disability insurance, and to life insurance through standard underwriting practices: denying coverage, or offering more expensive and more limited (substandard) coverage, to those who have a disease or are at higher risk of contracting it in the future, as determined by various tests, or medical records, or other predictors of risk, sometimes including medical examinations. One justification for these practices would be that they are necessary for the economic viability of insurance markets, protecting insurers against adverse selection. But risks to this defense are evident at least in the case of medical insurance in a climate in which many people think exclusions and risk rating are unfair. The risk is that people resent it when profits are more important than access to health care services; this resentment might increase antipathy toward a system of private insurance.

Because of these risks, it is not surprising that some insurers tried to seize higher moral ground with a position in defense of such a practice. The contention is that it is actuarially unfair, and therefore morally unfair, to those at low risk when insurers do not exclude those at high risk from insurance pools. Thus the hybrid term "actuarial fairness," widely used in the literature, expresses the moral judgment that fair underwriting practices must reflect the division of people according to actuarially accurate determination of their risks. This is the argument from actuarial fairness. It is intended to defend insurers against the claim of unfairness even in the case of medical insurance; if it works in this case, it seems to establish a moral argument for the uniform function thesis.

The concept of actuarial fairness could be assigned a purely descriptive as opposed to normative content in the kind of risk management insurance market that we discussed above. Saying that a premium is actuarially fair would mean only that it reflects the actuarial risks the purchaser faces, that it is actuarially accurate. In keeping with this descriptive view, insurers might claim that a properly functioning insurance market would tend to price insurance in ways that reflect actual (or known) risk levels of the insured.

The appeal to actuarial fairness that we find in the insurance literature goes beyond this purely descriptive content, however, and carries the implication that actuarially accurate underwriting practices are also morally fair or just. One way to defend such a claim would be to say that whatever prices (or exclusionary practices) occur in a properly functioning insurance market are themselves fair. The claim might derive from a general view about free exchanges: whatever exchanges people freely make in free markets should count as morally acceptable outcomes.

Without explicitly appealing to this more general position, insurers may be committed to it. In any case, they defend standard underwriting practices by claiming that insurance is founded on the principle that policy holders with the same expected risk of loss should be treated equally. Specifically, it will be unfair to those at low risk if they are made to pay higher premiums necessary to cover the costs of including those at high risk. Insurers assert that they have an obligation to refuse to underwrite those at high risk as part of the standard risk pool. If an efficient market would lead to market prices that reflect risks, insurers are saying they have an obligation to make sure their markets work efficiently.

The argument from actuarial fairness confuses actuarial fairness with moral fairness or just distribution. These are different notions: actuarial fairness is neither a necessary nor a sufficient condition for moral fairness or justice in an insurance scheme, especially in a health insurance scheme. To forge the link between fairness and actuarial fairness presupposes that individuals are entitled to benefit from their individual differences, especially their different risks for disease and disability. This presupposition is not only highly controversial, it is false. Without it, however, insurers cannot ultimately defend the fairness of prices that emerge in an efficient market where knowledge about risks is sufficient to produce stratification of risk pools.

To go from the merely descriptive notion of actuarial fairness, which has no justificatory force, to the moral claim about fairness in the insurers' argument, we must add some moral assumptions. Specifically, we have to add the strong assumption that individuals should be free to pursue the economic advantage that derives from their individual traits, including their proneness to disease and disability. The strong assumption might be used in a position that echoes some recent work on distributive justice: individual differences—any individual differences— constitute some of an individual's personal assets; people should be free to, indeed, are entitled to, gain advantages from their personal assets; social arrangements will be just only if they respect such liberties and entitlements; and specifically, individuals are entitled to have markets, including medical insurance markets, structured in such a way that they can pursue the advantages that can derive from their personal assets.

This skeletal concept can be elaborated, and its strong assumption can be defended (or attacked) in quite different ways within different theories of justice. For example, Nozick's (1977) libertarianism begins with certain assumptions about property rights and the degree to which some liberties, such as the liberty to exchange one's marketable abilities or traits for personal advantage, must be respected even in the face of what many take to be overriding social goals. In this view, actuarially unfair schemes confiscate property without consent. Other political philosophers claim that just arrangements are the result of a bargain made by rational people who want to divide the benefits of mutual cooperation. In this view, bargainers who have initial advantages in assets would accept only social arrangements that retain their relative advantages. As a result, bargainers might hold that just arrangements would preserve the advantages of those at low risk of disease through insurance markets that use standard underwriting practices.

An important objection to both libertarian and bargaining approaches is that the significant inequalities such theories justify can be traced back to initial inequalities for which there is little moral justification. To avoid this problem, Rawls (1999) imagined a "hypothetical contract" made by "free" and "equal" moral agents who are kept from knowing anything about their individual traits; they must select principles of justice that would work to everyone's advantage, including those who are worst off. Just which individual differences should be allowed to yield individual advantage thus becomes a matter for deliberation within the theory of justice, not a starting point for it. We now need a reason why this model for selecting principles is fair to all people and why we should count its outcome as justified, since we can no longer claim it is justified by appealing to the interests of actual property holders or bargainers (Rawls 1999).

The debate about the relevance of individual differences to the just distributions of social goods touches on deep issues about equality that lie at the heart of the conflict between alternative approaches to constructing and justifying theories of justice. Showing that the strong assumption about individual differences is deeply controversial at the level of the theory of justice is obviously not a refutation of the argument from actuarial fairness. Still, we now have good reason not to accept the assumption without a convincing reason.

As it stands, the strong assumption is much too strong, for it is inconsistent with other things we believe. Some individual differences are ones we clearly think should not be allowed to yield advantage or disadvantage for reasons of justice or fairness. Legislation in the United States established a legal framework to reinforce these views about justice. For example, race or gender should not become a basis for advantage or disadvantage in the distribution of rights, liberties, opportunities, or economic gain, even though each trait carries with it market advantage and disadvantage. Thus we reject, in its most general form, the view that all individual differences can be a moral basis for advantage or disadvantage.

Although we agree that race and gender are clearly unacceptable bases for advantage, less agreement surrounds how to treat other individual differences. We allow talents and skills, for example, to play a role in the generation of inequalities, and yet we tax those with the most highly rewarded talents and skills to provide help to those who lack them, at least to some extent (although not to the extent that the worst off are made as well-off as possible, as Rawls would have it). How much inequality we allow is controversial in practice just as it is in theory.

Some people, such as Nozick, think that individuals are entitled to derive whatever advantages the market allows from their talents and skills, and they view income redistribution as an unjustifiable tax on talents and skills. Others, such as Rawls, maintain that talents and skills such as intelligence and manual dexterity are results of a "natural lottery." Thus it is a matter of luck, not dessert, who enjoys family and social structures that encourage traits of character, such as diligence, necessary to refine one's basic talents. In this view, redistributive schemes are a morally obligatory form of social insurance that protects us all from bearing excessive burdens if we turn out to be among those who are worst off with regard to marketable talents and skills (Arneson 1989; Cohen 1989).

Even among philosophers who want to treat talents and skills as individual assets, only the strictest libertarians treat health status differences merely as unfortunate variations and believe that no social obligation exists to correct for the relative advantages and disadvantages caused by disease or disability. The design of health care systems throughout most of the world rests on rejection of the view that individuals should have the opportunity to gain economic advantage from differences in their health risks. Despite variations in how these societies distribute the premium and tax burdens of financing universal health care insurance, the mixed system of the United States is nearly alone in allowing the degree of risks to play such a role. Far from being a self-evident or intuitively obvious moral principle, the strong version of actuarial fairness is widely rejected, both in theory and practice.

Two further points about the practice of insurers and society strengthen the claim that we do not in fact treat actuarial fairness as a basic principle of distributive justice. If insurers thought it were such a basic principle, we might expect that they would try to develop and use all possible information about variations in risk among insureds. But they use information about risks only when it is in their economic interest to do so. For example, in marketing, it is not cost effective for insurers to engage in extensive medical underwriting, involving medical testing, for small amounts of life insurance, say under $100,000. In effect, the principle actually underlying practice is that we are entitled to benefit from our differences only if the market makes it worth while for insurers to provide such benefits.

This market-based entitlement can be construed as a principle of fairness only if we think the market is a fair procedure for drawing all the distinctions we want to make. But, and this is the second point, we do not trust the market to draw fair distinctions in this regard. We override appeals to actuarial fairness for many reasons in both medical and non-medical insurance contexts; we do so both for reasons of justice and for other reasons of social policy. For example, even in markets where no general social obligation is thought to make security against loss available to all, such as fire or theft insurance, it is generally recognized that certain underwriting practices are unacceptable forms of discrimination. Thus "red-lining" whole geographical areas was thought to contribute to the economic decline of neighborhoods and to "racial tipping" and "white flight," and that particular underwriting practice was condemned in the late 1970s as unacceptable. (A "red line" was drawn around a particular geographical area and its largely minority residents were excluded from insurance or mortgages.) No one questioned, however, the utility of red-lining as a (rough) device allowing insurers to predict their risks of loss. The point is that consideration of justice and social policy overruled the advantage of insurers of what hitherto had been standard underwriting practice.

Similarly, unisex rating, in the case of employee contributions and benefit pay-outs from employee benefits plans, is a rejection of an actuarially fair and efficient method of underwriting and pricing groups at different risks. Here too we override standard underwriting practice because we give more importance to a principle of distributive justice assuring equal treatment of women who have been the traditional targets of discrimination. Some states, recognizing the importance of access to health insurance coverage, established insurance pools that guarantee no one is deemed uninsurable because of prior medical condition or high-risk classification. Because such pools are often funded by premiums paid by low-risk individuals, we simply have an enforced subsidy from those at low risk to those at high risk, overriding concerns about actuarial fairness. Similarly, many states require high-risk drivers to be insured, setting up special pools or rate regulations, subsidizing high-risk drivers to make sure no one has to encounter uninsured drivers. Here our social interest in guaranteeing a public good (the reduced risk of encountering an uninsured driver) is allowed to overrule otherwise sound (and actuarially fair) underwriting practices that would have denied these drivers insurance.

Practices in these examples show that we do not believe that actuarial fairness is a basic requirement of justice. If it were, we would not override consideration of it for many reasons of social policy, which we do. We do not wholly trust insurance markets to draw distinctions between those occasions when actuarial fairness is acceptable—morally fair—and when it is not.

The argument from actuarial fairness, had we accepted it, might have made consideration of differences in the social function of types of insurance irrelevant. Since its premises are deeply controversial, and since we do not accept its implications in our social practices, we return to the strategy we articulated earlier.

Medical Insurance and Equality of Opportunity

The reason for rejecting the view that health insurance must be structured so that individuals can derive benefits from their differences in medical risks is compelling. To be sure, health care does many things for people: it extends life, reduces suffering, provides information and assurance, and in other ways improves quality of life. Nevertheless, it has one general function of overriding importance for purposes of justice: it maintains, restores, or compensates for the loss of (in short, protects) functioning that is normal for a member of our species.

Normal functioning is a crucial determinant of opportunities open to an individual, since disease or disability shrink the range of opportunities that would otherwise have been available to someone with particular talents and skills in a given society. Since justice requires that we protect fair equality of opportunity for individuals in a society, it requires that we design health care institutions, including their method of financing, so that they protect opportunity as well as possible within reasonable limits on resources. Specifically, justice requires that there be no financial barriers to access to care, and that the system allocate its limited resources so that they work effectively to protect normal functioning and thus fair equality of opportunity.

In fact, we have a rough way to assess the importance of particular health care services, namely, by their effect on the normal opportunity range. Since protecting equality of opportunity is a general social obligation, such as protecting basic liberties, all must share the burden for doing so; there can be no free riders. Moreover, other considerations of distributive justice imply that contributions toward this collective obligation should reflect ability to pay. A general theory of justice that includes a strong principle protecting fair equality of opportunity will be able to incorporate my account of justice and health care.

The view I have been sketching involves rejecting the argument from actuarial fairness. A health care system is just provided that it protects fair equality of opportunity. By permitting risk exclusions, our system fails to protect equal opportunity, since access to care depends on ability to pay. By permitting risk rating, our system requires that the sick pay more for health care rather than financing a collective obligation by ability to pay. Therefore, the way these underwriting practices try to meet social obligations regarding access to health care is to institute a universal, compulsory national health insurance scheme. Under social insurance schemes, prior medical conditions and risk classification cannot serve as bases for underwriting or pricing insurance coverage. Rather, because society acts on its obligation to meet all reasonable health care needs, within limits on resources, subsidies will come from the well to the ill and from low-risk to high-risk individuals, as well as from the rich to the poor. The social insurance scheme thus requires what a private market for health insurance would condemn as actuarially unfair. This point is independent of whether the scheme includes a sector with private insurance. German and Dutch systems, for example, have many private insurers, but they are prohibited from using our standard underwriting practices, and insurance is compulsory, preventing free riders.

From the perspective of a private insurer in our mixed system, one insisting exclusively on the risk-management function of insurance, denying coverage to those at high risk seems completely unproblematic. (You can't buy fire insurance once the engines are on the way.) But this perspective is persuasive only if the central function of health insurance is risk management. Since health insurance has a different social function, protecting equality of opportunity by guaranteeing access to an appropriate array of medical services, a clear mismatch exists between it and standard underwriting practices (and the voluntariness of participation in insurance). A just, purely public system thus leaves no room for the notion of actuarial fairness.

Ironically, a just but mixed public and private health insurance system makes actuarial fairness a largely illusory, perhaps even deceptive, notion. Suppose that high-risk individuals, for example, those with a history of serious heart disease, are excluded from private insurance in a mixed insurance system, for the reasons we noted earlier. Since the system is just, however, these people will not be left uninsured, as many are in the United States today. They will be covered by public insurance or by legally mandated high-risk pools subsidized by premiums from private insurance. Those lower-risk individuals left in private schemes might think that actuarial fairness has protected them from higher premiums. But here is where their savings are largely illusory. Their premiums will either cross-subsidize to some degree high-risk individuals who are insured in special high-risk pools, or their taxes will cover the costs of insuring high-risk individuals through public schemes. Their actual insurance premiums are thus their private ones plus the share of their taxes that goes to public insurance. The main point of principle in a just, mixed system is this: low-risk individuals still share the burden of financing the health risks of high-risk individuals.

Fairness requires that these risks be shared, the contrary of the conclusion from the argument from actuarial fairness that they not be. Of course, risks must be shared by everyone. In effect, health risks are not treated as economic assets and liabilities for the individual.

One clarification regarding risk rating is necessary. In a system based on progressive taxation, such as the Canadian system, the primary form of health care subsidy is from richer to poorer participants, although it will also be true that the well subsidize the ill. The well subsidize the ill because there is no risk rating within income (or tax contribution) levels. Such a system embodies, in effect, two principles of distributive justice: that ability to pay should govern contributions, not coverage, and that we must share the burden of health risks and we are not entitled to benefit economically from having better health.

In a system that retains private insurance and that relies primarily on premium-based financing, community rating means that some poorer but well individuals will subsidize some richer but sicker individuals. This system is clearly not ideal. It abandons the distributive principle that is present in the tax-based system; namely, that ability to pay should determine contributions, since everyone pays the same premium. In this nonideal setting, community rating appears to make the situation worse, adding to the regressivity. But the question is, what alternative to community rating is being proposed? If it is to drop premium-based financing and to endorse progressively tax-based financing, the system would clearly be more just. But if the alternative is to retain premium-based financing and to add risk rating, the system would be less just, for it would also reject the principle that health risks are not to be viewed as economic assets from which we can gain or lose as the case may be. Paradoxically, despite its regressivity, a community-rated premium system is preferable to one that is both regressively financed and makes the sick bear a greater economic burden for their condition (Daniels et al. 1996). A fuller defense of community rating in this nonideal situation would require showing that it is more important to establish the importance of well and ill sharing risks together than it is to insist on full progressivity of financing.

The genome project will generate information that insurers in our mixed system will want to use in standard underwriting practices, not because they are greedy but because they respond to the incentives we have built into the design of our system. The argument I have offered says that such uses will make our system less fair, more unjust. But the problem is not that new information emerges from the genome project. In a national health insurance scheme that prohibited our morally unacceptable underwriting practices, information about risks would not be used to exclude people from treatment but to improve counseling, education, and treatment. It is not availability of information that is bad, but how our system encourages insurers to use it. If we fail to correct the more basic injustice in the health care system, singling out information from the genome project for special treatment would itself seem arbitrary. The problem must be corrected at its source—the design of our health care system—not simply where a new symptom of the injustice arises.

The Social Functions of Disability and Life Insurance

Medical insurance is not simply an instrument for individual risk management; it has the additional social function of protecting equality of opportunity by assuring everyone access to necessary medical services. Therefore, justice requires that we not permit risk exclusions or risk rating, or actuarial fairness, to constitute barriers to insurance coverage and thus to access to care.

Is there an analogous argument for disability and life insurance both of which are more discretionary than medical insurance? Or is individual risk management the sole important function of these forms of insurance? To find out, we must examine what social functions are served by disability and life insurance. We can then decide whether we have obligations regarding these functions that imply we should abandon or modify standard underwriting practices in these cases as well. It should also be kept in mind that group disability and group life insurance are not medically underwritten, although they are subject to experience rating. The focus of our discussion, as in the case of health insurance, is on the section of these insurance markets where medical underwriting is widely practiced.

Both disability and life insurance serve more than one purpose or function. Thus, life insurance provides not only income support but a chance to preserve an estate. Similarly, disability insurance may sometimes include special medical or rehabilitation benefits in addition to income support. I will not discuss the medical benefits of disability insurance, as the same considerations would apply to them that apply to medical insurance. Indeed, in most national health care insurance systems that provide universal, comprehensive coverage, it is not necessary to include medical benefits, including physical and mental rehabilitation benefits, within disability coverage at all. These benefits appear in our system only because we lack universal, comprehensive medical insurance.

Private disability insurance may also provide resources—income well above the level of social disability benefits—that an individual can use for job retraining. They may allow an individual to avoid the negative market effects of losing some capabilities through a disability. Like medical services, such occupational refitting preserves the range of opportunities open to an individual, compensating for loss of some by substituting others. This type of disability benefit would be of value to individuals at all income and education levels within the system. To the extent that it would discharge our social obligation to protect equality of opportunity, it should not be seen simply as an individual instrument of risk management, something that individuals who prefer a certain kind of security should be able to buy if they can afford it. It is a benefit we have a social obligation to make sure is available to people.

If we have this social obligation to provide for job retraining after development of disabilities, we must not allow medical underwriting, including genetic underwriting, to interfere with it. We cannot, however, eliminate medical underwriting without making insurance compulsory. Nevertheless, job retraining is not the typical use of disability benefits, and we should not conclude that all disability insurance should be managed in the way appropriate for this component. At best, the argument shows only that our public system of disability insurance should have such a component.

We return to the primary function of disability insurance, which is income support aimed at countering short- or long-term disruption of employment. This is one function that disability insurance shares with life insurance, for a central function of life insurance is to protect families against the permanent income loss that results from early death. To what extent should we see this key function of both kinds of insurance as a simple instrument of individual risk management? To what extent might social obligations, or at least very strong social interest provide some forms of income preservation above the social minimum already provided by public disability insurance? Disability and life insurance can be linked because they share this same function of income preservation. Life insurance, however, also has other functions, such as estate preservation, protection of businesses, and protection against loan indebtedness, which introduce quite different issues. So we are not treating these types of insurance as equivalent, only similar with regard to the important function of income support.

Private disability insurance provides a level of income support that is aimed at preserving a significant percentage, usually 60% to 66%, of the income an individual would have had without disability. This level of protection is considerably above that provided by the public safety net of social disability insurance, which is means tested, yet it is set well below full replacement for several reasons. First, if premiums are paid for in after-tax dollars, disability benefits are tax free. Second, to discourage moral hazard, there is reason to want replacement for income to fall below predisability income. Third, public insurance (SSDI) benefits are not means tested and are not affected by the presence of other disability income.

The benefit of private disability coverage is clear: individuals or their families do not have to survive at the low level of income provided by public insurance. Moreover, some families will not have to decrease their assets to the point at which they are eligible for means-tested income support. Family stability is preserved: housing and education plans may be sustained, and resources are available for job retraining, if necessary. In the homogeneity view, these benefits show why prudent agents reasonably averse to risks prefer to pay modest premiums out of disposable income to obtain such economic security. This same rationale holds true for purchasers of life insurance seeking to preserve the economic integrity of their families.

Social benefits also derive from individual ones. By providing their own insurance, such individuals clearly spare the social insurance scheme the need to cover them through other welfare schemes. Private insurance schemes have other public effects: less uncertainty within higher-income families; more stability to child rearing and education plans; and more stability to family life, housing, and other fundamental elements of modern life. Given these important benefits, it is quite reasonable for society to take steps to make sure markets for such private insurance work well and are stable. Protecting the markets generally means permitting medical underwriting for risks of disability and premature death.

So far, this societal interest falls well short of a social obligation to assure that these individuals can secure their desired level of income protection, regardless of their levels of risk. We have nothing matching the argument from equality of opportunity that was key to showing why medical insurance should not be governed by the risk-management view. Indeed, we seem to have a paradigm case of what the risk-management view presumes: if certain individuals want to buy greater economic security at a price, let them do so, and it may be in society's interests to assure stable markets within which this can occur. It is reasonable and fair to use medical underwriting, including genetic information, if that is what it takes to make that market stable.

One serious obstacle to an analogy between the medical case and the issue of income support in disability and life insurance is that incomes vary enormously. It is quite unclear why people interested in preserving a significant proportion of their low or middle-level incomes should be interested in sharing risks with someone whose needs for income support are an order of magnitude higher.

Is there really a common interest across income groups, as there is in protecting our ability to sustain normal functioning? We must separate the problem of risk sharing from the problem of insuring different income levels in order to meet this objection. Suppose that premiums in a private disability or life insurance scheme reflect the level of benefits: higher-income people would pay higher premiums than lower-income people since they would be given high levels of income support. The question remains whether people at each income level have some obligation, or at least important common interest, to share risks, avoiding medical underwriting. For example, they might agree that they have a common interest in preserving legitimate expectations about standard of living, even when they have disabilities. For all people to agree that their expectations about standard of living were legitimate, they might have to agree that income inequalities in the society formed part of a scheme of inequalities that was just, and that these inequalities operated against a background that assured equality of opportunity. I doubt that we could agree on this, but let us suppose a situation in which we would. Then what everyone supports is a system that provides the chance for all to live in accordance with their reasonable expectations about standard of living.

So far we have described a scheme in which a common interest exists across income groups in preserving income during periods of disability or in the event of premature death, and this can be accomplished without compelling lower-income people to cross-subsidize higher income levels for higher-income people; although high-income benefits would be available to those at lower income levels if the appropriate premium level were paid. The issue that remains is whether medical underwriting, including genetic underwriting, should be permitted. This question is equivalent to the next one: given that premium levels will reflect benefit levels, should they also reflect expected benefit levels, since expected benefit levels will reflect risks? In medical insurance, the same arguments that weigh against making those who are sickest pay more for actual use of services also weigh against making those at highest risk pay more for their expected benefits. In admitting that those who will receive high income-support benefits should pay more for them, have we admitted that medical underwriting has no moral objection? Let us divide the problem by income groups.

Do high-income people interested in securing high levels of income support during disability through disability or life insurance have an obligation to pool their risks? If some people are at low risk because of their medical history and genotype, do they have an obligation to cross-subsidize the income-support benefits of other high-income people who are at higher risk? In the case of medical insurance, we held that the obligation to protect equality of opportunity compelled risk sharing and cross-subsidies. But it is implausible to believe in a social obligation to preserve expectations about standard of living that are enjoyed by the best-off groups in society. Rather, it seems reasonable to expect them to use their high incomes when not disabled to buy this protection for themselves or their families in the event of their premature death.

In the absence of such an obligation, we have no reason to compel those at lower risk to support those at higher risk. This position is less compelling for lower-income people, say those whose family income is below the median level. We might be more concerned that those who faced higher medical risks of disability or early death might find it too difficult to protect their legitimate expectations regarding standard of living because their premiums would be significantly higher. But wanting to protect those at greater risk requires imposing higher costs on those at lower risk. Do we have adequate justification for doing so here?

A necessary condition for keeping a private disability insurance system viable without medical underwriting is that it be made a compulsory insurance scheme. This is the claim of private insurers who insist that no one would write disability insurance without medical underwriting unless participation were compulsory. But establishing compulsory private disability insurance to cover people above the social safety net provided by public disability insurance up to some ceiling, such as median family income, is equivalent to raising the social safety net.

What this shows is that we cannot insist that genetic information, or medical information more generally, should not be used in underwriting disability insurance unless we are willing to demand that level of coverage as if it were a social safety net. We might be willing to distinguish a socially required minimal safety net, provided by public insurance, from the somewhat higher socially desired adequate safety net, provided by compulsory private disability insurance. We might think of the public level as a requirement of justice and the private level as a beneficial social policy that we are justified in making compulsory, even if it is not a requirement of justice. In doing so, we would be acknowledging that such insurance has a social function—keeping people at an adequate standard of living—sufficiently compelling to view it as more than just an individual instrument of risk management. This does not insist on that higher level of safety net; instead, it shows what kind of system would be necessary to make the income-support function of disability insurance immune to medical underwriting. We remind the reader that the analysis applies both to disability insurance and to modest levels of life insurance.

Some Policy Implications

The issue of medical underwriting in life insurance has been addressed in other countries. In the 1990s both The Netherlands and Canada made policy recommendations to prohibit medical underwriting, including genetic underwriting, for life insurance benefits below a ceiling. The Canadian Privacy Commission recommended that for life insurance policies under $100,000 there be no medical underwriting. In The Netherlands, a five-year trial was introduced in which no genetic information was permitted in underwriting insurance policies less than 200,000 guilders (approximately $100,000). Subsequently, numerous countries enacted a range of laws dealing with the use of genetic information in life insurance underwriting (see chapter 8).

Rothstein (1993) suggested two further restrictions on policies that set ceilings on coverage without the consideration of genetic information. First, it would be important to restrict eligibility for nonunderwritten insurance to an aggregate equal to the ceiling value. No one should be able to collect on several such policies. Second, it is justifiable to insist on a reasonable waiting period, say one year or even two, before the benefit of a policy is in place (Rothstein 1993). (This practice is not permitted under present New York State law.) Otherwise, people near death, who had never contributed to an insurance scheme, would unfairly benefit from contributions of others. It should be remembered that nothing in this proposal would change the existing practice of age rating life insurance premiums.

Whether the policy recommended by the Dutch, as amended by Rothstein, would put insurers at great risk is an empirical question. We may learn something from the Dutch experience, but the Dutch and United States insurance markets differ in important ways. In The Netherlands, life insurance rates are fixed by regulation, so price competition is minimal. The market has features of a cartel. An underwriting prohibition may then have different effects from a similar one in the United States. Any policy we introduced of this sort should also be subject to a clear trial period with careful monitoring. It is not in our interest to undermine a system that works well, as evidenced by the fact that currently 88% of applicants for life insurance are offered preferred or standard rates and nearly 70% of United States families carry some level of life insurance. It is also possible to alter the benefit levels that are eligible for protection against underwriting. Since many insurers find it cost ineffective to do significant underwriting for small policies, the policy implications of this proposal may be much less significant than they seem.

One final qualification regarding policy: both Canada and The Netherlands provide much more generous systems of health, disability, and income support than we do in the United States. Their social safety net is considerably higher and tighter in all dimensions than ours. Against that background, where the gap between the social safety net and the private life insurance net is not too great, it is quite reasonable for them to insulate from underwriting reasonably generous life insurance protection. The discrepancy between our private insurance protection—if we assured people access to some level of it without underwriting—and our public safety net might seem unjustifiable, even embarrassing. It would seem more important to raise the public safety net. Some, however, might not find such a gap embarrassing because they hold particular views about the justifiability of a strong division between public and private responsibility. In the absence of a belief in limiting the public sphere, the gap seems hard to justify.

Is Genetic Information Different?

Throughout this chapter, I have drawn no distinction between standard medical underwriting and the use of genetic information or genetic screening to enhance standard underwriting. Is genetic information different? Does it warrant special treatment?

Several differences are typically pointed to in contrasting genetic screening for underwriting purposes with other forms of medical underwriting. Although some of them raise important worries, they do not seem to indicate a fundamental difference in kind, at least one that is relevant to considerations of fairness.

Rothstein (1993) raised the notion that genetic diseases, at least single-gene disorders, are conditions an individual could do nothing to avoid, in contrast to medical conditions to which an individual may contribute through lifestyle choices. This seems irrelevant to the debate about medical underwriting, the point of which is to determine risks, not to ascribe responsibility for them. (Some believe we do not owe people insurance for conditions they bring on themselves, but the object of medical underwriting is not to distinguish self-induced from other medical risks but to identify all medical risks.)

If we set aside the claim of irrelevance and insist on responsibility, the result may end up cutting two ways. Suppose we are considering the case of insurance for children whose genetic diseases or disorders could have been avoided, say by genetic screening and elective abortion, but parents chose to avoid such screening and had the children anyway. The fact is that the children are not responsible for the disorder, the parents are, at least in part; and perhaps even more directly responsible than other people are for their lifestyle choices.

A stigma may affect families, and not just individuals, in the case of genetic disorders. This means that privacy concerns affect not just the individual, but whole families in a way that may not arise with other medical conditions.

Individuals may be comfortable accepting some risks to their own privacy when they insure themselves, but fear imposing those risks on family members where genetic testing is involved. This concern reinforces the importance of protecting privacy and confidentiality, but it does not constitute a reason for exempting genetic information from underwriting practices. Family histories raise genetic issues informally, so we must already protect privacy through adequate regulation. If medical information can be protected against privacy violations, so too can genetic information. The priority must be to develop adequate protections for all underwriting, not selectively to pick out some elements for special exclusion.

Some genetic conditions, and hence screening for them, may differentially affect sensitive racial or ethnic groups. Policies that have a different negative effect by race, for example, will be highly controversial and may run afoul of antidiscrimination legislation. The same point raises more general historical associations with eugenics (Buchanan et al. 2000). These considerations place the burden of proof on those who would invoke genetic information for underwriting purposes (Rothstein 1993).

Suppose Rothstein is right. Can this burden of proof be met? It seems it can be met in two ways: show the risk of adverse selection because individuals seek this information for their own purposes, and show that adverse selection can be avoided by demanding that genetic information be available to insurers whenever it is available to individuals. Assuming privacy concerns can be satisfied, the fact that individuals want the information themselves shows that the bugaboo of the eugenics movement does not make the information taboo.

The burden of proof would be heavier if insurers wanted to initiate significant amounts of genetic screening themselves, independent of evidence that individuals had the results of such tests. So far, it seems unlikely that insurers would want to introduce such programs. The reasons are economic, not moral.

The economics go heavily against insurer-initiated genetic screening. The only circumstance in which such an effort would seem likely involves several very strong assumptions:

1. Testing would have to be relatively inexpensive and highly predictive of significantly increased risks.

2. For that to be true, conditions for which screening is done would have to be relatively common, and the difference in risk levels between those who test positive and those who do not would have to be quite high (or the screening would very likely be cost ineffective).

3. People would not be likely to obtain this information for their own purposes (or else the information would be available to insurers without screening).

4. It would have to be possible to offer the product at much lower cost to a sizeable market as a result of the testing.

5. Testing would have to avoid a significant effect on sensitive groups, such as races.

Some of these assumptions cut against each other: if a test were highly predictive and involved a common condition, many people would seek to have it, and insurers would not have to perform screening for it.

Together these considerations suggest that the use of genetic information rather than other information for medical underwriting is not so essential that it warrants special restrictions on insurance underwriting. Instead, policy efforts should focus on guaranteeing adequate privacy controls for all uses of medical information.

Summary

The social function of a particular type of insurance is an important factor in determining the justice or fairness of risk rating. The argument from actuarial fairness, had we accepted it, might have made consideration of differences in the social function of different types of insurance irrelevant; however, the analysis presented reveals the significance of this social function. The view I have sketched involves rejecting the argument from actuarial fairness in the context of health insurance.

A health care system is just provided that it protects fair equality of opportunity. By permitting risk exclusions, our system fails to protect equal opportunity, since access to care depends on ability to pay. By permitting risk rating, our system requires that the sick pay more for health care rather than financing a collective obligation by ability to pay. Therefore, these underwriting practices undercut fairness rather than assure that our system is just. The social obligation for assuring income support as in disability and life insurance is somewhat less compelling.

What this suggests is that we cannot insist that genetic information, or medical information more generally, should not be used in underwriting disability or life insurance unless we are willing to insist on that level of coverage as if it were a social safety net. We might be willing to distinguish a socially required minimal safety net, provided by public insurance, from the somewhat higher socially desired adequate safety net, provided by compulsory private disability insurance. We might think of the public level as a requirement of justice and the private level as a beneficial social policy that we are justified in making compulsory, even if it is not a requirement of justice. In doing so, we would be acknowledging a social function of such insurance—keeping people at an adequate standard of living—sufficiently compelling to view it as more than just an individual instrument of risk management. I have not argued for that higher level of safety net; instead, I have tried to show what would be needed to make the income-support function of disability or life insurance immune to medical underwriting. The analysis applies both to disability insurance and to modest levels of life insurance.

In conclusion, the type of insurance and the individual and social purpose it serves may dictate the type of information that should or should not be used by insurers in making coverage decisions. Nevertheless, development of a policy concerning the use of genetic information in assessing risk should not distinguish genetic from other medical information. Rather, consideration should be given to assuring and enhancing the privacy protections provided to individuals and their families.

Notes

1. An earlier version of this chapter was originally drafted for a project on the implications of the Human Genome Project for insurance directed by Alex Capron. I owe considerable thanks to Mark Rothstein for extensive effort editing the original draft to make it suitable for this volume.

2. The argument in this section was presented with a focus more specifically on HIV in Daniels, N., Seeking Fair Treatment: From the AIDS Epidemic to National Health Reform. New York: Oxford University Press (1995).

References

American Academy of Actuaries, Issue Brief: Genetic Information and Voluntary Life Insurance. (1998), available at www.actuary.org/pdf/life/genet.pdf.

Arneson, R., "Equality and Equal Opportunity for Welfare," Philosophical Studies 56: 77–93 (1989).

Buchanan, A. et al., From Chance to Choice: Genetics and Justice. Cambridge: Cambridge University Press (2002).

Cohen, G. A., "On the Currency of Egalitarian Justice," Ethics 99: 906–944 (1989).

Daniels, N. et al., Benchmarks of Fairness for Health Care Reform. New York: Oxford University Press (1996).

Institute of Medicine, National Academy of Sciences, Care Without Coverage: Too Little, Too Late. Washington, D.C.: National Academy Press (2002).

Nozick, R., Anarchy, State, and Utopia. New York: Basic Books (1977).

Rawls, J., A Theory of Justice. Cambridge, MA: Belknap Press (rev. ed. 1999).

Rothstein, M., "Genetics, Insurance, and the Ethics of Genetic Counseling," in Molecular Genetic Medicine vol. 3, T. Friedmann, ed. San Diego: Academic Press (1993).

7

Perspectives of Consumers and Genetics Professionals

Wendy R. Uhlmann and Sharon F. Terry

Adam, age 46, requested genetic testing for Huntington disease. His mother was diagnosed with the disease in her forties and died at age 51. His 50-year-old brother was diagnosed with Huntington disease in his thirties. Adam understood that his risk was theoretically 50%; however, since he was without symptoms at age 46, the risk was decreased to approximately 37%. Adam wanted to be tested because he had two teenage children and was applying for life insurance so that his family would be taken care of in the event something happened to him. At the time of his clinic visit, two different companies had denied him life insurance. Adam wanted to prove to the companies that he did not have the Huntington disease gene mutation. If a mutation was identified, his attitude was that at least the life insurers would have a legitimate reason for denying him coverage.

—Patient seen in the University of Michigan Medical Genetics Clinic

Until recently, genetic tests were available primarily for genetic conditions affecting a small segment of the population. With rapid advances based on the Human Genome Project, they will be available for common conditions, including cancer, heart disease, and diabetes. Increasing numbers of predictive tests will be done on healthy individuals to determine future risk for genetic conditions. Such advances hold great promise for preventive health care and treatment, yet they also have the potential for causing stigmatization and discrimination depending on how genetic information is used by insurers and employers.

The Insurance Dilemma

It may be reasonable for a society to require that healthy people subsidize the health insurance or health care of those who are ill, but it is unreasonable to require that healthy people subsidize the estate building of people with current or future lethal illnesses.

—Mark A. Rothstein (1993, p. 168)

Simply stated, if life expectancy is much shorter than anticipated, purchasing life insurance at standard rates is the world's best financial investment.
—Robert J. Pokorski (1997, p. 208)

Consumers in the United States feel that health insurance, and to some extent life insurance, is a right. Individuals interviewed by the Genetic Alliance expressed a sense of indignation, even when they were symptomatic, that insurers would not cover them or give them the lowest premiums (unpublished data). They expected to be able to obtain life insurance, and could not imagine that not only would they be affected by a genetic condition, but that they would also have to pay higher premiums or be denied coverage altogether.

The life insurance system in the United States is risk based, meaning that the applicant's health status and behaviors, as determined by an insurance provider and quantified by an actuarial table, are the major indicators for whether one acquires insurance and at what premium. Therefore, life insurance is based on both demographic and personal risk. In such a system, it is important to assess risk accurately and equitably. Genetic risk is still largely indeterminable, however, particularly because environment plays a large role in the expression and variability of disease. Life insurers uniformly raise rates or deny insurance to individuals who participate in high-risk activities, such as rock climbing or sky diving, even though the chance of death or disability from these activities is very low. In contrast, a child of a parent with an autosomal dominant condition has a 50% risk of being affected; perhaps this is enough cause, in a risk-based system, to apply high-risk rates to the child. "Even if society can accept the need for a life insurer to charge a higher premium based on life expectancy, ethical considerations in pricing genetic risk are more complex and troubling because the risk of disease is present at conception and is often inescapable" (Nolan 2002, p. 195).

Life insurers are concerned that individuals at risk for genetic conditions will seek to purchase large policies at standard rates without disclosing genetic information. Consumers fear that genetic information will be used by insurance companies, including life insurers, to increase premiums or deny or limit coverage. Other consumer concerns are at follows:

• Insurers will force consumers to have genetic tests to determine eligibility for insurance coverage, even when they would prefer not to know their genetic status.

• Insurers' access will adversely affect the privacy and confidentiality of genetic information.

• Insurers' use of genetic information will prevent consumers' participation in research studies.

• Insurers' use of genetic information will prevent consumers from proceeding with genetic and medical tests and finding out information that would benefit their health care and life decisions.

Several surveys (National Center for Genome Resources 1996; Lapham et al. 1996) document consumer concerns about insurers' use of genetic test results and the impact these concerns have on their decisions to have genetic testing. A widely cited study by the Genetic Alliance (called the Alliance of Genetic Support Groups at the time of the study) and HuGEM (Human Genome Education Model Project II) with Georgetown University Child Development Center, found that 9% of respondents declined genetic testing, 18% withheld genetic information from insurers, and 17% withheld genetic information from employers because of fear of discrimination (Lapham et al. 1996). These results were based on a survey, with follow-up telephone interviews, of 332 individuals with one or more family member with a genetic disorder.

From a purely economic standpoint, consumers have no incentive to share positive genetic test results with life insurance companies, because these results would likely adversely affect their coverage. On the other hand, it is to their benefit to share negative results, because this information could result in lower premiums, particularly if family history had placed the consumer in a high-risk category. Insurance companies face the opposite problem. According to Pokorski (1997), "Insurers are confronted with a dilemma. They are being asked to credit all favorable genetic information so that more people can obtain insurance coverage and at the same time, they are told that unfavorable genetic tests must be ignored" (p. 208). Genetic factors cannot be ignored in underwriting, however, as this would result in individuals of known risk being placed in the wrong group, and would violate the principle of equity (Zimmerman 1998).

The very nature of what constitutes genetic information is also unclear. Increasingly, lines are becoming blurred between genetic and nongenetic information and between genetic and other medical tests. Genetic tests are not the only sources of genetic information. Clinical examinations and other medical tests (radiographs, scans, echocardiograms, cholesterol levels) are also frequently used to diagnose a genetic condition. Family history remains one of the most informative sources.

The confusion over what constitutes genetic information was evident in a study of state insurance commissioners (McEwen et al. 1992). Whereas few state commissioners indicated that such information was used in underwriting, review of application forms from major life insurance companies showed that many contained questions about family history and required tests (e.g., blood tests for cholesterol). Such questions and test results provide genetic information. Using a broad definition, therefore, genetic information has always been a part of medical information; however, a distinction, real or not, is being pressed as a result of the availability of molecular genetic testing. For insurance determinations to be based on genetic information, the definition must be clarified, as well as its relationship to medical information. In addition, the extent and timing of insurer access to this information must be established.

Who Is at Risk for Genetic Discrimination?

Everyone is at risk for having a condition that has an underlying genetic component. However, some individuals are at risk of genetic discrimination who will not develop the condition that causes the discrimination (Natowicz et al. 1992; Bornstein 1996). The following are examples:

• Individuals who are carriers of certain recessive or X-linked genetic conditions but will remain asymptomatic (e.g., cystic fibrosis, Tay-Sachs disease, Duchenne muscular dystrophy).

• Individuals with genetic conditions that can be treated before the onset of symptoms or have symptoms managed so that they have no significant health problems and lifespan is normal (e.g., phenylketonuria, hemochromatosis).

• Individuals with gene mutations that make them susceptible to adverse health, but only if exposed to specific environmental agents (e.g., malignant hyperthermia, glucose-6-phosphate dehydrogenase deficiency).

• Individuals who have genetic polymorphisms that are not known to cause disease (e.g., blood group polymorphisms).
• Relatives of individuals with genetic conditions. Depending on the pattern of inheritance, they may not even be at risk.

All of us carry gene mutations for a handful of genetic conditions that follow an autosomal recessive pattern of inheritance. Being a carrier is usually of no adverse health consequence, and it is only when both parents are carriers for the same autosomal recessive condition that they have a 25% risk for having an affected child.

Other genetic conditions are inherited in an autosomal dominant manner, which confers a 50% risk for each child of an affected or carrier parent. Nevertheless, because of reduced penetrance, not all genotypes are expressed as disease phenotypes. Individuals who have gene mutations with reduced penetrance for genetic conditions (e.g., hereditary breast cancer, hereditary nonpolyposis colon cancer) may never develop the condition but could transmit the gene mutation to a child who does. Individuals may also have gene mutations that increase the risk for a multifactorial or complex disease, but they may not necessarily develop the disease due to other modifying genes or different environmental factors (putative genes for diabetes, cancers, heart disease, Alzheimer disease).

Some genetic conditions have variable expressivity, such that even if the individual is affected, he or she may have no significant problems and have a normal lifespan (neurofibromatosis, myotonic dystrophy, Charcot-Marie-Tooth syndrome). Low et al. (1998) found that individuals at risk for genetic discrimination include healthy carriers of autosomal recessive or X-linked conditions, noncarriers of genes for late-onset disorders, and parents of children whose condition was the result of a spontaneous mutation.

Studies Documenting Genetic Discrimination

I have been denied life insurance, although I am 21 and quite healthy, because I put down on the application that my father has Huntington disease. I don't have any signs of the disease, nor have I ever been tested for it. And I don't want to fight it—I am afraid of what will happen to my health insurance, though I don't think they are from the same company.
—Woman respondent in Genetic Alliance survey (2001)

One might ask if fear of genetic discrimination is widespread, why do so few studies document it? The reasons are that genetic testing has been available to only a small segment of the population, individuals are afraid to come forward, individuals do not know whom to approach with insurance complaints, and people have little legal redress.

One of the earliest studies purporting to document genetic discrimination was conducted by Billings et al. (1992). In the study, 1,119 professionals in clinical genetics, genetic counseling, disability medicine, pediatrics, and social services in New England were directly solicited to provide cases of possible genetic discrimination. This solicitation for cases was also published in the *American Journal of Human Genetics* and newsletters of organizations of individuals with genetic conditions, including Friedreich ataxia, Charcot-Marie-Tooth syndrome, and muscular dystrophy.

Only forty-two responses were received over seven months and thirteen (31%) had to be excluded either because they did not meet the study's criteria for genetic discrimination or they provided insufficient information. Most of the twenty-nine remaining responses were submitted by individuals who saw the study announcement in newsletters of organizations of individuals with genetic conditions. These responses included forty-one separate incidents of possible discrimination: thirty-two insurance, seven employment, and two adoption. Although the authors cited the case of a woman with Charcot-Marie-Tooth syndrome (a nonfatal, highly variable neuromuscular condition) who was denied life insurance several times, they did not indicate how many of the cases involved life insurance. Specifically, respondents had problems obtaining desired coverage; new, renewed, or upgraded policies were frequently unobtainable, even when applicants were asymptomatic. These problems arose primarily when they altered existing policies due to relocation or changes of employers.

Although this study received widespread publicity for purportedly documenting genetic discrimination, in reality, the few cited cases actually provided evidence for the opposite view that insurance discrimination resulting from use of genetic information is not a significant concern. Despite surveying over 1,100 health care professionals who would have had information on thousands of patients, only forty-two individuals felt strongly enough about their insurers' decisions to reply to the survey (Reilly 1999). Hundreds of thousands of life insurance policies would have been issued in that region during the seven-month survey period (Lowden 1992).

The few cases of discrimination were by written report only and none was researched to make sure the claim was valid. Clayton (1999) suggested that there were few cases of discrimination ascertained in the study because respondents had to take the time to write their stories, thus lowering the response rate (Clayton and Rothstein 1999). The lack of responses on the part of health care providers was attributed to the fact that these professionals have little time for surveys because they spend time each week advocating for patients with insurance companies. Based on the limited information provided, Lowden (1992, p. 903) wrote that some "bad decisions were made" and "may represent mistakes in judgment based on lack of information," but did not believe that the decisions represent typical insurance practice.

In Dorothy Wertz's 1992 study (published in 1997), of 1084 genetic service provider respondents who were board-certified by the American Board of Medical Genetics and/or full members of the National Society of Genetic Counselors, 237 had a patient who was refused life insurance because of carrier status and 237 had an asymptomatic patient who was refused life insurance because of a genetic predisposition (Wertz 1997). The genetic service providers had a median of fourteen years' experience in genetics and a median of six patients per week. Of 473 patients from 12 genetics clinics, 5% reported that they or a member of their family had been denied life insurance because of a genetic disability or disease. These cases of discrimination were by report only and were not confirmed. Based on the results, Wertz (1997) postulated that genetic discrimination exists, but is rare, and it is also possible that health care providers do not query patients specifically about insurance issues. These results "suggest that fears about genetic discrimination may be exaggerated" (Wertz 1997, p. 468).

The Billings et al. (1992) survey served as a pilot study for the larger study on genetic discrimination conducted by Geller et al. (1996), which sent surveys in 1992–1993 to 27,790 individuals on the mailing lists of the Huntington Disease Society of America, Hemochromatosis Research Foundation, National M.P.S. (mucopolysaccharidoses) Foundation, and PKU (phenylketonuria) Clinic at Boston Children's Hospital (Geller et al.

1996). Of 917 respondents, 455 (49.6%) indicated that they had experienced genetic discrimination, 437 (47.7%) had not, and 25 (2.7%) had ambiguous answers that could not be specifically classified. Overall, 623 respondents (67.9%) had or were at risk for Huntington disease, and 276 (44.3%) indicated that they had experienced genetic discrimination. Whereas 47.7% of overall respondents stated that they had not experienced such discrimination, many noted that they had adopted strategies to minimize this risk and ensure that others would not learn their genetic information.

The article did not include a breakdown of each type of genetic discrimination so it is not known how many cases involved life insurance. The cases of genetic discrimination were by report only and not confirmed. The response rate was low (less than 5%) and the number of individuals reporting discrimination represented less than 2% of those who were surveyed.

The investigators conducted follow-up scripted telephone interviews with 206 of 917 respondents who were willing to be contacted and whose survey responses met study criteria for genetic discrimination, one of which was that they were asymptomatic. In cases involving health and life insurance, the investigators noted discrimination against individuals who were asymptomatic; consideration of a genetic diagnosis as a pre-existing condition, which resulted in different treatment of asymptomatic individuals and family members; loss of insurability by relatives of a person with a presumed genetic disease; and failure of some group plans to provide coverage for qualified individuals with a genetic diagnosis.

Two cases of life insurance discrimination were cited. One case involved a healthy twenty-four-year-old woman with a family history of Huntington disease whose application for life insurance was denied because she had not had genetic testing to determine her carrier status. Kass (1997) also noted that there have been instances where insurance is denied to children who have a parent with Huntington disease, unless the child is tested and has a negative result. In the other case, an unaffected child whose sibling had Hurler syndrome was denied coverage.

The Genetic Alliance, a coalition of more than 300 patient advocacy groups, conducted two studies on genetic discrimination in insurance. Participants for the first one were recruited through postings in its monthly bulletin and by a mailing sent to 101 directors of support groups, representing approximately 585,800 members. The response rate was less than 1%. Although respondents were willing to complete anonymous surveys, far fewer agreed to be interviewed. Twenty-five percent of respondents reported that they or a family member had been denied life insurance (Lapham et al. 1996). In addition, many stated that they had never applied for life insurance because they assumed they would be denied coverage. No breakdown was provided as to the number of respondents who were affected with a genetic condition (which could account for the high percentage who were denied life insurance) versus those who were unaffected. Cases of reported genetic discrimination were not confirmed.

The second study was conducted in 2001 (unpublished data). Of 234 respondents, 54 indicated that they had experienced life insurance discrimination (refusal or higher rates); however, 34 were symptomatic for a genetic condition, thus negating their claim of discrimination. Some respondents indicated that they were denied life insurance based on family history and then told that they could reapply after undergoing genetic testing. Conditions included adult polycystic kidney disease, Marfan syndrome, Huntington disease, hereditary cancers (breast, ovarian, multiple endocrine neoplasia), Alzheimer disease, hemochromatosis, α_1-antitrypsin deficiency, hyperoxaluria, Turner syndrome, and pseudoxanthoma elasticum.

During follow-up telephone interviews, confirmation of discrimination was not obtained for thirteen of twenty asymptomatic individuals. Of seven who described discrimination, five were reportedly discriminated against because a family member (parent, 3; brother, 1; son, 1) was diagnosed with a hereditary genetic condition, although they themselves had no symptoms and did not have genetic testing for the condition. A thirty-eight-year-old woman revealed during a job interview that her father had Alzheimer disease. She did so because her resume included antidiscrimination activities and her future boss asked about her involvement in these activities. When she was hired, she was told she was denied enrollment for life insurance because of her father's Alzheimer disease.

Two individuals were asymptomatic, but tested positive for a presumably disease-causing mutation. One man was denied life insurance by five different companies because he tested positive for a mutation for Marfan syndrome. He was asymptomatic and was tested only because his symptomatic brother was diagnosed with the disorder. His brother did have life insurance, however, because he obtained the policy before onset of symptoms and subsequent diagnosis.

A review of genetic discrimination studies concluded that "little evidence supports the widespread fear that people who undergo genetic tests to determine whether they are at increased risk for developing a serious disorder face a significant risk of genetic discrimination" (Reilly 1999, p. 106).

Consumers' Handling of Insurance Problems

It is not known how many individuals, when denied desired coverage, contact their insurers to learn the reasons for this decision or take other steps to pursue the matter. In the 2001 Genetic Alliance survey, two of seven individuals claiming discrimination were unwilling to appeal the decision to deny insurance for fear of losing their job and potential effects on their health insurance, even though a different company provided it. Reilly (1999) was unable to identify a single legal case in which consumers sued insurers alleging genetic discrimination in underwriting.

The Medical Information Bureau, Inc. (MIB) maintains a national database and provides information to insurance companies about medical histories of applicants obtained from the application process. Whereas it is possible to review these records and request corrections, only ten (18%) of fifty-five respondents knew about the existence of the MIB and none asked to review their records. Insurance complaints can be raised with state insurance commissions. Only nineteen (33%) of fifty-eight respondents knew about these commissions, and most thought that their purview was limited to auto insurance. Even those who knew about these regulatory agencies often did not press their grievances, with some stating that they perceived they had little chance of success (Geller et al. 1996), and others were fearful of disclosing personal information to state commissioners (Geller et al. 1993). Complaints about genetic discrimination are also less likely to be reported by the poor, the uneducated, and foreign nationals who are unlikely to know whom to contact and how to "work the system."

A nationwide survey of insurance commissioners found that only two of thirty-nine state commissioner respondents had formally received complaints from applicants or policy holders about alleged genetic discrimination by life insurers (McEwen et al. 1992). The total number of complaints was fewer than seven, and they were being investigated at the time the article was written.

Does Genetic Discrimination by Life Insurers Occur?

I have a 36-year old patient with very mild myotonic dystrophy (only clinical signs are his hands get weak after he uses them for very prolonged periods of time) identified after a distant relative had a child with the congenital form. He is trying to get life insurance but is encountering some resistance.

—Posting on National Society of Genetic Counselors listserv (August 2002)

A mother who has a newborn with Klinefelter's syndrome recently tried to get life insurance for her son and this was denied.

—Posting on National Society of Genetic Counselors listserv (July 2002)

[Mild myotonic dystrophy and Klinefelter syndrome are not associated with increased morbidity and mortality.]

A healthy woman in her late 20s tested positive for a BRCA1 mutation, which predisposes her to hereditary breast-ovarian cancer. She had a prophylactic double mastectomy and hysterectomy, which made her risk for cancer lower than that of the general population. Subsequently, when she applied for life insurance and reported her recent surgeries, the insurance company said that it would need to review her medical records. Her request for life insurance was denied due to information contained in her medical records that specifically included her BRCA1 genetic test results. Staff from the National Human Genome Research Institute became involved in the case. Not only did she receive a life insurance policy but it was issued at one of their lowest rates. She stated, "Enlightment won the battle over ignorance."

—Abstracted from a posting on the Genetic Alliance listserv (May 2002)

When exploring whether genetic discrimination occurred as a result of ignorance by the institution or as a result of policy, evidence was found for both, although no statistics were provided (Geller et al. 1996). It was specifically noted that there were agents in a branch office who were unaware that their company policy stated that individuals with asymptomatic hemochromatosis should not be denied a policy.

Data from a study in the United Kingdom provide evidence of unjustified genetic discrimination by insurers (Low et al. 1998). The study included 264 unaffected carriers of recessive disorders, 59 healthy noncarriers of late-onset disorders, and 210 noncarrier parents of children with disorders due to spontaneous mutation. Of these 533 individuals who did not represent an adverse actuarial risk, 71 (13%) had experienced problems obtaining insurance, which they believe was due to their genetic status. These problems included outright refusal (35%), higher premiums (47%), unnecessary medical examinations (13%), and other difficulties (51%). In a comparison group drawn from a sample of the general public who answered questions on applying for life insurance as part of an omnibus survey, only 39 (5%) of 736 had problems obtaining life insurance.

Some insurers seemed to be erroneously treating carriers of genetic conditions as if they had the actual disease (Low et al. 1998). Eleven percent (28/264) of unaffected carriers of recessive disorders (e.g., cystic fibrosis, Duchenne muscular dystrophy, conditions that arise in childhood) had problems obtaining life insurance, as did 46% (27/59) of healthy noncarriers of autosomal dominant disorders (e.g., Huntington disease, myotonic dystrophy). In addition, 82% of healthy noncarriers of autosomal dominant disorders were charged higher premiums. Many conditions are genetic but not inherited, and arise due to a spontaneous mutation. Some 8% (16/210) of noncarrier parents of children with disorders due to spontaneous mutation experienced difficulty obtaining insurance.

Whereas this study provides evidence of genetic discrimination by insurers, it is limited because it did not research and verify each reported case of discrimination. It is possible that other causative factors were not determined that posed an actuarial risk.

Strategies for Minimizing Genetic Discrimination

I advise all prospective presymptomatic patients to settle life, health, disability and long term care issues before having testing.
—Posting on National Society of Genetic Counselors listserv (April 2002)

Genetic counselors must be cautious about the problem of adverse selection. A vigorous position of patient advocacy might lead a practitioner to tolerate or even advise a patient on how to maximize the benefits of genetic testing without risk of losing insurance or paying higher premiums. Others would oppose such a position, not only because of the deception involved if important information is withheld from insurers, but because they advocate cooperation between insurers and providers as the best way to achieve fair and reasonable policies in the long run.

—American Society of Human Genetics (1995, p. 330)

Potential strategies can be used both by health care professionals and by patients to minimize risks for genetic discrimination. For health care professionals:

• Advise patients before genetic testing of potential risks for genetic discrimination (insurance, employment).
• Advise patients to "load up" on health, life, and long-term disability insurance before genetic testing.
• Allow patients to self-pay to avoid submission of health insurance claims for genetic services.
• Suggest/allow patients to be tested anonymously or under an assumed name.
• Keep genetic test results in a "shadow chart," separate from office or hospital charts and inaccessible to third-party payers.
• Advise patients' physicians not to place genetic test results in medical records.
• Provide limited chart documentation regarding the purpose of the clinic visit and where test results are sent.
• Submit false reports regarding the individual's genetic condition to insurance companies.

(Rothstein 1993; Hall and Rich 2000)

For patients,

• Purchase insurance policies before genetic testing.
• Self-pay for genetic tests.
• Provide incorrect name or have testing done anonymously.
• Withhold or provide partial relevant medical or family history information to health care providers and insurers.
• Provide incorrect medical or family history information to health care providers and insurers.
• Decline genetic testing and avoid situations in which genetic information could be used against them.

(Rothstein 1993; Geller 1996; Billings et al. 1992)

In a 1997 study by Hoyle to which 272 genetic counselors responded, 36.9% indicated that they might advise patients to purchase insurance before testing, 81.1% would allow patients to self-pay, 37.6% would permit anonymous testing, 25.3% would provide partial reports to third parties, and 57.4% would maintain shadow charts. In addition, 48.3% would discuss available resources regarding the use of genetic information with patients, including state and federal laws. However, 61.3% would inform patients that nondisclosure of genetic information to insurers could be considered fraud. In 1997, the National Society of Genetic Counselors, the professional organization for genetic counselors, had 1,599 members (National Society of Genetic Counselors 1997) of whom survey respondents represented approximately 17%. Although this study provides some insight as to how genetic counselors approach concerns about genetic discrimination with patients, large-scale studies of health care professionals, particularly genetics specialists, should be conducted to determine comprehensively the extent to which strategies listed above are used.

Several respondents of one study withheld or "forgot" to mention potentially important family or medical history information to insurers, employers, or physicians (Billings et al. 1992). Others stated that insurance agents suggested they provide incomplete or dishonest information on insurance forms.

In a 1993 article, Rothstein considered whether it was ethical for health care professionals to advise individuals on how to avoid genetic discrimination, applying the strategies listed in Table 7.3:

Advise Patients about Risks for Genetic Discrimination

Advising patients before testing about potential risks for genetic discrimination is completely ethical. "There can be no real informed consent if the individual is not told that he or she may become unemployable or uninsurable as a result of the test" and "the failure to provide such information might even be considered actionable negligence" (Rothstein 1993, p. 173). Guidelines for predictive testing for Huntington disease and cancer susceptibility specifically state that patients should be informed of these risks (International Huntington Association and World Federation of Neurology 1994; American Society of Clinical Oncology Subcommittee on Genetic Testing for Cancer Susceptibility 1996; Geller et al. 1997). Genetics professional societies also issued position papers stating that the subject should be discussed with patients (McKinnon et al. 1997; American Society of Human Genetics ad Hoc Committee on

Genetic Testing/Insurance Issues 1995). Informed consent forms for genetic testing sometimes included mention that results could affect coverage (Durfy et al. 1998; Hall and Rich 2000). A risk exists, however, that unless disclosures are made in a balanced, careful way, patients will have exaggerated and unreasonable fears of genetic discrimination. This, in turn, could lead them to adopt some of the strategies listed above.

Allow Patients to Self-Pay for Genetic Services

It is not illegal or unethical to allow patients to pay for their genetic testing or other medical services. For a number of reasons patients may prefer to pay in cash, such as to avoid being sent an insurance claim that would be received or seen by a spouse or other family members (Rothstein 1993). Whereas self-paying for genetic testing means that the insurer initially would not know about the testing, if the patient is seen for other medical indications that are submitted for coverage, the insurer would then have access to the patient's medical record, including documentation of genetic test results.

Offer Anonymous Testing

Anonymous testing is available regarding HIV status because of concerns about stigmatization and discrimination (Rothstein 1993), which are also risks for genetic testing. Some favor anonymous genetic counseling and testing (Mehlman et al. 1996), whereas others do not (Uhlmann et al. 1996; Clayton and Rothstein 1996). They contend that accurate family and medical history information is critical to providing genetic counseling, including determining whether genetic testing is indicated, which test should be ordered, and accurately interpreting results.

Limit Chart Documentation and Access to Medical Information

Discretionary documentation of indications for clinic visits is one strategy used by genetic counselors to maintain secrecy of genetic information (Hall and Rich 2000). For example, a visit for genetic testing would be noted as screening for cancer. Another method involved not reporting results to the referring physician unless specifically requested to do so by the patient, and advising the physician not to record the results in the medical chart. Genetic clinics may maintain shadow charts separate from hospital medical records. However, whereas "shadow charts" could limit insurers' ability to access this information, they would legally be considered part of the patient's hospital medical record. It would be unethical to keep shadow charts that would be inaccessible to insurers (Rothstein 1993). In addition, it could compromise the integrity of patients' medical information. Furthermore, failure on the part of the physician to disclose pertinent medical information, if detected by the insurer, could result in denial of the claim.

Submit False Reports
Submitting false reports would be unethical and could result in charges of fraud if discovered.

Advise Patients to "Load Up on Insurance" before Testing
This advice presents an ethical quandary as it could be viewed as a component of informing patients about potential risks of genetic discrimination. It would also allow individuals to obtain insurance for which they later may not qualify and to obtain it at standard rates. According to Rothstein (1993), the advice to "load up on insurance" would be tantamount to advising the individual to lie on the medical questionnaire when applying for life insurance, essentially, providing them with the last opportunity to mislead an insurer. Thus the "genetic service provider would be, in effect, aiding and abetting the commission of fraud" (Rothstein 1993). However, if the advice is given in the context that one must not withhold or provide dishonest answers to medical questions, it would be less ethically problematic. At the University of Michigan Medical Genetics Clinic, it has been our approach to inform patients to make sure that they have insurance coverage that they need before testing, but not to advise them specifically to load up on insurance.

Patient Strategies
Strategies that patients can utilize to minimize the potential risks for genetic discrimination were also listed earlier on p. 159. Providing false information, withholding information, or providing partial disclosure to insurers puts the patient at risk for policy cancellation or for legal prosecution for fraud. It is not legally clear as to how asymptomatic individuals who have had a positive predictive or presymptomatic genetic test should answer questions on an insurance application (Kass 1997). The

individual is not symptomatic and, even though he or she has had a positive test, this does not necessarily mean that symptoms will occur.

Consumers at high risk for genetic disease could purchase ten $25,000 life insurance policies, which would not be scrutinized as closely as buying a single $250,000 policy (Zoler 1991, cited in Pokorski 1997). Nevertheless, insurers often ask applicants about other policies they have or for which they have applied. As more genetic tests are marketed directly to consumers, this will provide a means for individuals to obtain genetic information without physicians' or insurers' knowledge. Some predict that in the future, consumers would have the option of private genetic screening through home test kits, mail-order kits, and walk-in testing at shopping malls (Andrews et al. 1994, cited in Pokorski 1997).

Do High-Risk Consumers Load Up on Life Insurance?

Insurers have a major concern that individuals who are at risk for a genetic condition with increased morbidity or mortality will buy an excessive amount of insurance. Few studies have examined actual occurrence of this possibility. Geller et al. (1996) reported in their study that several individuals at risk for Huntington disease indicated that they had either attempted to buy life insurance or increase their coverage at the time that they learned of their at-risk status or when they experienced onset of symptoms (Geller et al. 1996).

One study examined whether individuals known to be at high risk for a genetic condition would capitalize on this information and purchase more life insurance was conducted by (Zick et al. 2000). This was part of a larger National Cancer Institute longitudinal study evaluating behavioral and psychosocial consequences of genetic testing. Women from a large, hereditary cancer kindred were studied over a one-year period. Those who underwent research genetic testing to determine whether they were carriers of a BRCA1 mutation were compared regarding their purchase of life insurance policies with 177 women in the general population who had not had genetic testing, and had at least one first- or second-degree relative with breast or ovarian cancer. Women with a BRCA1 mutation in the kindred had an 88% combined risk of developing either breast or ovarian cancer by age 70. Theoretically, women who learned that they were at high risk could purchase large life insurance policies at standard rates, as insurers would not have access to genetic test results obtained as part of a research study.

The women selected for this study had to have no personal cancer history and had to carry life insurance that was not paid entirely by their employer. There were 105 women in this kindred, age 18 to 55 years, the prime age range for purchasing life insurance policies, that met these criteria; 28 (27%) tested positive and 77 (73%) tested negative for a BRCA1 gene mutation. Some of them had participated in earlier research that led to the discovery of the BRCA1 gene, and may have suspected that they carried a gene mutation before being tested in the later study. The authors concluded that neither family history, testing status, nor participation in early BRCA1 research had an effect on demand for life insurance. No differences were found in the number of life insurance policies and total amount of coverage between women in the study kindred and the sample from the general population. Therefore, women who knew that they were carriers of a BRCA1 mutation and had a high risk for cancer did not capitalize on this knowledge by purchasing more life insurance.

The authors cautioned against extrapolating their results to the general population, as their study involved a rather homogeneous group of women, most of whom were active members of the Church of Jesus Christ of Latter Day Saints. Of this study group, only 28 women had a BRCA1 mutation. The authors postulated that the women did not purchase more life insurance because the genetic test results only confirmed the risk they and their insurers had already surmised based on their family histories. It is also possible that the study duration was too short, and addressing health care issues rather than life insurance would likely have been a higher priority for these women after learning their test results.

Perceptions of Genetics Professionals

A study of genetic counselors specializing in cancer genetics was conducted to ascertain how they would approach genetic testing if they themselves were at 50% risk of carrying a mutation for either BRCA1 or BRCA2 (hereditary breast or ovarian cancer) or hereditary nonpolyposis colon cancer (HNPCC) (Matloff et al. 2000). Of 163 genetic counselors responding to a survey, 85% indicated that they would pursue genetic testing for BRCA1 and BRCA2 and 91% would test for HNPCC. The two main reasons why they would not test for BRCA1 or BRCA2 were fear of genetic discrimination and because they did not think the results would affect their medical management at that time. In addition, 67.9% of counselors indicated that they would not submit charges for genetic testing to insurance companies, and 25.8% would use an alias for testing because of fear of discrimination. Those who were concerned about genetic discrimination specifically feared that their future insurability might be jeopardized, feared discrimination against their children, and did not believe existing laws were adequate to protect them in this regard. Whereas the number of counselors who would self-pay or use an alias was significant, it is important to note that these results do not necessarily reflect the views of the profession overall. In 1998, there were 1718 members of the National Society of Genetic Counselors (National Society of Genetic Counselors 1998), and therefore survey respondents represented less than 10% of this total.

In another study, interviews were conducted with 29 experienced genetic counselors-medical geneticists about genetic discrimination (Hall and Rich 2000). Of these, 92% reported that patients seeking presymptomatic genetic testing had concerns about the potential for insurance discrimination, with most (67%) having a high level of concern. Whereas health insurance was the major concern (59%), 18% of respondents noted that patients were concerned about life insurance coverage. Furthermore, 38.1% (8/21) stated that discrimination concerns are a major barrier to testing for adult patients.

In the same study, 84% of genetic counselors-geneticists noted that they routinely discuss the risk of genetic discrimination with individuals considering genetic testing. The risk was largely raised with adults and rarely with pediatric or prenatal patients. In the authors' review of informed consent forms for adult-onset genetic conditions, seven (64%) of eleven forms cited insurance discrimination as a potential risk of genetic testing, whereas only one (7%) of fourteen forms for prenatal, pediatric, or generic genetic conditions included this risk. Most counselors reported spending on average approximately fifteen minutes of a one- to two-hour session discussing genetic discrimination. According to sixteen of twenty-two counselors, when they discussed the subject they informed patients that the actual frequency of discrimination was low, that the risks applied to specific types of insurance, and that some legal protections were available. Counselors also attempted to reassure patients by describing various confidentiality measures in place to protect medical information.

Genetic counselors and geneticists reported that most patients' awareness of the potential for genetic discrimination came from the news media and television. Concern was particularly evident for patients considering genetic testing for Huntington disease. Counselors attributed this concern to the Huntington's Disease Society of America making patients aware of this possibility as well as patients' own experiences with affected family members.

Another survey of genetic counselors also found that concern about potential use of genetic information by insurers or employers was greater for adults than for pediatric or prenatal patients (Hoyle et al. 1997). Of 272 respondents, the potential use of genetic information was often or always a concern when counseling patients in cancer genetics (92.1%), neurogenetics (82.7%), adult genetics (80.2%), pediatric genetics (35.7%), and prenatal genetics (18.8%). However, overall, 50.6% of respondents indicated that patients rarely or never expressed concern about the potential use of genetic information by third parties, and 44.5% reported that privacy of that information was rarely or never a concern. When queried about the counseling they provided three months before completing the survey, many respondents stated that they never or rarely discussed the implications of genetic information with patients for life insurance (44.4%), health insurance (33.3%), disability insurance (58.3%), or employability (45.2%).

Problems with Insurers' Use of Genetic Tests

Despite the introduction of innumerable screening, diagnostic and therapeutic technologies over the past century, the percentage of people who have been able to obtain life insurance has in fact remained stable or increased.
—Robert J. Pokorski (1995, pp. 13–14)

From a scientific standpoint, the predictive nature of genetic tests combined with the fact that genetics is not destiny creates difficulty interpreting genetic tests. Testing for many genetic conditions is not yet standard of care and the tests themselves are far from standard. Many tests are costly and have a low detection rate. Often a gene mutation has to be identified in an affected individual before at-risk family members can undergo testing. The significance and implications of results may be uncertain, unknown, or not interpretable. The detected gene mutation may not cause disease but could be a common polymorphism or rare sequence variant. Even if the mutation does cause disease, several variables can influence its clinical expression. Particularly for rare conditions, it may be years before sufficient data are collected and the significance of test results is fully understood.

The Need for Genetics Expertise in Ordering and Interpreting Genetic Tests

It is increasingly a challenge for geneticists and genetic counselors to keep up with rapid advances in the field. Determining whether a test is indicated, which one to order, which laboratory to use, and how to interpret the results requires genetics expertise. A test may be relatively straightforward to perform in the laboratory but limited in clinical application or complex to interpret. Dewar et al. (1992) note that insurers often overestimate individual risk if penetrance and variable expressivity are not taken into consideration when using genetic information. Medical directors of insurance companies "need assistance in maintaining a current knowledge base in new, rapidly changing fields such as genetics" and "without help [from the genetics community], they will make some poor decisions" (Lowden 1992, p. 903).

Peter S. Harper, a well-respected geneticist, believes that the risk for adverse selection due to individuals knowing genetic test results that are unknown to insurers is extremely limited. Tests for autosomal recessive conditions, X-linked conditions, and chromosomal abnormalities will be of little relevance to life insurers because many of these conditions have onset in childhood, with early mortality and major morbidity (Harper 1997). Results for autosomal dominant conditions such as Huntington disease would be of interest to life insurers, but many conditions are rare, with tests ordered because of a family history or because a person is symptomatic. Multifactorial conditions are the most common in the general population and therefore of most relevance to life insurers.

However, because they involve a combination of genetic and environmental factors and are not just due to a single gene, tests for them will be difficult to develop and complex to interpret.

For hereditary cancer syndromes and other conditions, genetic test results may significantly improve prognosis by allowing for early diagnosis (Harper 1997). The possibility of early diagnosis or treatment could directly benefit the insurance industry by reducing mortality, and new customers could be generated from individuals receiving normal test results. The bottom line is that "life insurance companies could, with little loss, forego the use of or knowledge of genetic test results other than in exceptional situations, and that the industry could indeed benefit from avoiding the need to assess an increasing volume of complex and largely irrelevant data" (Harper 1997, p. 1066).

Family history remains one of the most informative "genetic tests." No cost is involved and no blood sample is required. "Questions about parents' or siblings' disease, time from diagnosis and death will provide the insurer with information that can predict the individual's risk of dying at a young age or become ill more effectively than results from genetic predisposition tests" (Norum and Tranebjaerg 2000, p. 190).

Summary

Most diseases are not a person's fault or under one's control. Exempting genetic diseases or information from risk classification would be equivalent to saying that applicants with all other disorders were responsible for their illnesses.
—Robert J. Pokorski (1995, p. 14)

Genetic tests offer individuals the chance to learn whether or not they are affected or at risk for a genetic condition. This information could have significant implications for health care and life decisions for the individual and relatives. Results may affect preventive options, surveillance, treatment, and care. Even when results indicate a genetic condition for which no treatment exists, they may be of great benefit in life decisions. They could bring great relief to individuals who find that they do not have or are not at risk for a genetic condition. However, consumers' fear of how results could be used by insurers may prevent them from experiencing these benefits. In addition, fear may prevent individuals from participating in research to enhance understanding and treatment of genetic conditions.

Every one of us has genetic alterations that predispose toward disease. We have no control over the genes that we inherit, and few genetic conditions are amenable to dietary or other interventions. It is clear from studies cited in this chapter that genetic discrimination does exist. Its frequency appears small, but it must be considered in the context that genetic testing has been available only to a small segment of the population. Studies conducted to date are largely based on patient reports. Larger, comprehensive studies are necessary to document the frequency of genetic discrimination and take the extra steps to investigate cases need to be investigated to confirm that discrimination actually occurred.

To say that life insurers cannot use genetic information or test results is impractical. Distinctions between genetic information and nongenetic information and genetic tests and medical tests are not clear-cut. Not only is what constitutes "genetic" not easily defined, it is so widely pervasive in medical records that it would be practically impossible to separate genetic information from other information. "Separate treatment increases the stigma attached to genetic conditions and lends legitimacy to genetic reductionism and determinism" (Rothstein and Anderlik 2001, p. 357). The number of genetic tests is only going to increase, and as they become part of routine medical care, they will find their way into use by the insurance industry. Unlike other medical tests that are the same regardless of which laboratory performs them, variability can be present in genetic tests. It may be years before data are sufficient to determine the laboratory and clinical accuracy of the tests and, given their complexity, great care is necessary in their use and interpretation. Therefore, it would be beneficial for both consumers and insurers if a fair approach could be worked out regarding use of genetic information to ensure that coverage remains widely available at affordable rates for all.

References

American Society of Clinical Oncology Subcommittee on Genetic Testing for Cancer Susceptibility, "Statement of the American Society of Clinical Oncology: Genetic Testing for Cancer Susceptibility," J. Clin. Oncol. 14: 1730–1736 (1996).

American Society of Human Genetics ad Hoc Committee on Genetic Testing/ Insurance Issues, "Background Statement: Genetic Testing and Insurance," Am. J. Hum. Genet. 56: 327–331 (1995).

Andrews, L. et al., eds., Assessing Genetic Risks: Implications for Health and Social Policy. Washington, DC: National Academy Press (1994).

Billings, P. R. et al., "Discrimination as a Consequence of Genetic Testing," Am. J. Hum. Genet. 50: 476–482 (1992).

Bornstein, R. A., "Genetic Discrimination, Insurability and Legislation: A Closing of the Legal Loopholes," J. Law Policy 4: 551–610 (1996).

Clayton, E. W., "Comments on Philip R. Reilly's 'Genetic Discrimination,'" in Genetic Testing and the Use of Information, C. Long, ed. Washington, D.C.: American Enterprise Institute (1999), pp. 134–138.

Clayton, E. W. and Rothstein, M. A., "Anonymous Genetic Testing: Reply to Mehlman et al." [letter], Am. J. Hum. Genet. 59: 1169–1170 (1996).

Dewar, M. A. et al., "Genetic Screening by Insurance Carriers," JAMA 267: 1207–1208 (1992).

Durfy, S. J. et al., "Testing for Inherited Susceptibility to Breast Cancer: A Survey of Informed Consent Forms for BRCA1 and BRCA2 Mutation Testing," Am. J. Med. Genet. 75: 82–87 (1998).

Geller, G. et al., "Genetic Testing for Susceptibility to Adult-onset Cancer: The Process and Content of Informed Consent," JAMA 277: 1467–1474 (1997).

Geller, L. N. et al., "Insurance Commissioners and Genetic Discrimination," Am. J. Hum. Genet. 52: 1018 (1993).

Geller, L. N., "Individual, Family, and Societal Dimensions of Genetic Discrimination: A Case Study Analysis," Science and Engineering Ethics 2: 71–88 (1996).

Hall, M. A. and Rich, S. S., "Patients' Fear of Genetic Discrimination by Health Insurers: The Impact of Legal Protections," Genet. Med. 2: 214–221 (2000).

Harper, P. S., "Genetic Testing, Life Insurance and Adverse Selection," Phil. Trans. R. Soc. London 352: 1063–1066 (1997).

Hoyle, C. L. et al., "Discussion of Genetic Discrimination Issues by Genetic Counselors and Their Clients," J. Genet. Counsel. 6: 455–456 (1997).

International Huntington Association and the World Federation of Neurology Research Group on Huntington's Chorea, "Guidelines for the Molecular Genetics Predictive Test in Huntington's Disease," Neurology 44: 1533–1536 (1994).

Kass, N. E., "The Implications of Genetic Testing for Health and Life Insurance," in Genetic Secrets: Protecting Privacy and Confidentiality in the Genetic Era, M. A. Rothstein, ed. New Haven, CT: Yale University Press (1997).

Lapham, E. V. et al., "Genetic Discrimination: Perspectives of Consumers," Science 274: 621–624 (1996).

Low, L. et al., "Genetic Discrimination in Life Insurance: Empirical Evidence from a Cross Sectional Survey of Genetic Support Groups in the United Kingdom," Br. Med. J. 317: 1632–1635 (1998).

Lowden, J. A., "Genetic Discrimination and Insurance Underwriting," Am. J. Hum. Genet. 51: 901–903 (1992).

Matloff, E. T. et al., "What Would You Do? Specialists' Perspectives on Cancer Genetic Testing, Prophylactic Surgery, and Insurance Discrimination," J. Clin. Oncol. 18: 2484–2492 (2000).

McEwen, J. E. et al., "A Survey of State Insurance Commissioners Concerning Genetic Testing and Life Insurance," Am. J. Hum. Genet. 51: 785–792 (1992).

McKinnon, W. C. et al., "Predisposition Genetic Testing for Late-onset Disorders in Adults: A Position Paper of the National Society of Genetic Counselors," JAMA 278: 1217–1220 (1997).

Mehlman, M. J. et al., "The Need for Anonymous Genetic Counseling and Testing," Am. J. Hum. Genet. 58: 393–397 (1996).

National Center for Genome Resources, National Survey of Public and Stakeholders' Attitudes and Awareness of Genetic Issues, www.ncgr.org/gpi/survey/Index.html (1996).

National Society of Genetic Counselors, Annual Report, Wallingford, Pa.: National Society of Genetic Counselors (1997).

National Society of Genetic Counselors, Annual Report, Wallingford, Pa.: National Society of Genetic Counselors (1998).

Natowicz, M. R. et al., "Genetic Discrimination and the Law," Am. J. Hum. Genet. 50: 465–475 (1992).

Nolan, W., "A Rational View of Insurance and Genetic Discrimination," Science 297: 195–196 (2002).

Norum, J. and Tranebjaerg, L., "Health, Life and Disability Insurance and Hereditary Risk for Breast or Colorectal Cancer," Acta Oncol. 39: 189–193 (2000).

Pokorski, R. J., "Genetic Information and Life Insurance," Nature 376: 13–14 (1995).

Pokorski, R. J., "Insurance Underwriting in the Genetic Era," Am. J. Hum. Genet. 60: 205–216 (1997).

Reilly, P. R., "Genetic Discrimination," in Genetic Testing and the Use of Information, C. Long, ed. Washington, DC: American Enterprise Institute (1999).

Rothstein, M. A., "Genetics, Insurance and the Ethics of Genetic Counseling," Mol. Genet. Med. 3: 159–177 (1993).

Rothstein, M. A. and Anderlik, M. R., "What Is Genetic Discrimination, and When and How Can It Be Prevented?," Genet. Med. 3: 354–358 (2001).

Uhlmann, W. R. et al., "Questioning the Need for Anonymous Genetic Counseling and Testing," Am. J. Hum. Genet. 59: 968–970 (1996).

Wertz, D. C., "Reports of 'Genetic Discrimination': A Survey of Clients and Providers," J. Genet. Counsel. l6: 467–468 (1997).

Zick, C. D. et al., "Genetic Testing, Adverse Selection and the Demand for Life Insurance," Am. J. Med. Genet. 93: 29–39 (2000).

Zimmerman, S. E., "The Use of Genetic Tests and Genetic Information by Life Insurance Companies: Does this Differ from the Use of Routine Medical Information?," Genetic Testing 2: 3–8 (1998).

Zoler, M. L., "Genetic Tests: Can We Afford the Answers?," Med. World News January: 32–37 (1991).

8

A Comparative International Overview

Bartha Maria Knoppers, Béatrice Godard, and Yann Joly

The possibility of using genetic information and testing in life insurance underwriting has stimulated legislative and policy discussion at all levels, international, regional, and national. Even in countries with universal health care, the debate on genetics and life insurance has included potential restrictions on the use of genetic information, since life insurance is closely linked to the acquisition of primary, modern socioeconomic goods (e.g., homes, cars, loans). In Europe, where for the most part universal health care systems are in place, the debate on life insurance is equally active: "Public anxiety focuses on two main areas: that people will be pressured into having unwanted genetic tests in order to obtain insurance, and that genetic testing will create an underclass of people ..." (Read 2002, p. 5). Life insurance appears to be a uniform need, closely linked as it is to family responsibilities. Thus, in many European countries access to it is seen as a basic socioeconomic good, a right, not a privilege. In contrast, the debate in the United States centers on genetics and access to health insurance. Hitherto, scant attention has been paid to issues surrounding life insurance per se.

Life insurance contracts rest on the principle of utmost good faith. This means that all relevant information known to the applicant must be declared. Selection among different risks allows the insurer to limit and rate the premium. To achieve this goal, the applicant must give all information requested by the insurer, and voluntary false declaration voids the contract.

In the insurance contract, rational, scientifically sound and empirically supported discrimination is permissible. Discrimination among risks is considered ethically problematic only where there is no sound actuarial basis for the manner in which the risks are classified, or individuals of the same risk class are treated differently.

Hence the more information available to the insurers the better, the more precise the discriminations the greater the actuarial fairness of the system. (Anderlik and Rothstein 2001)

It is common practice to ask applicants to fill out a personal and family history health questionnaire. Because life insurance is built on mutuality, risk spreading, and pooling, undeclared or false information leading to an assessment of risk that is not actuarially sound both affects the premium and skews the pool. Taking out a large policy at a favorable premium based on genetic information that is not shared with the insurer creates asymmetry of information known as adverse selection. If this practice becomes widespread, "then the whole of mutuality-based insurance collapses" (Read 2002, p. 4). The European Committee of Insurance (1998), referring to the importance of obtaining all relevant information pertaining to the risk, stated: "[T]o assess the risk in full knowledge of the facts, the insurer most dispose of the means to evaluate the components of the risks. The Committee is therefore opposed to any measure depriving insurers of relevant or significant information on the candidate's health." Finally, mutuality based systems should be distinguished from solidarity based schemes of universal health systems in Europe. The latter are usually compulsory with fixed rates set by the government.

The European Union imposes three principles: free circulation of tests, freedom to establish the enterprise, and freedom to offer services. Free circulation of genetic tests raises questions about their technical accuracy. Quality assurance is both for registration and for marketing. Another question is the relevance of such tests to life insurance. Free establishment requires states to welcome on their territory the insurance companies of other member states as registered and controlled by their original state. Any company can commercialize its products in the European Union market. However, in the life insurance industry, it is the law of the insured person's country that applies to the contract, not the law of the country of the insurer. This may foster either a narrower or broader vision in deciding what constitutes discrimination based on health reasons.

Even though several European organizations have clearly taken a stand against genetic discrimination, the position paper of the European Committee of Insurance of 1998 was not so categorical. On the one hand, as concerns the importance of being correctly informed on the state of health of a proposer (applicant), it states that "[a] questionnaire including a series of questions on the proposer's health [is routine and] no European insurer requires a genetic test." On the other hand it says, that "to assess the risk in full knowledge of the facts, the insurer must dispose of the means to evaluate the components of the risks. [The] CEA is therefore opposed to any measure depriving insurers of relevant or significant information on the candidate's health."

Finally, central to the debate is the definition of genetic information as distinct from other medical data. "Clear definitions of terms used in genetics, insurance and employment should be developed, so that different professions and their clients have a common understanding of the issues" (European Society of Human Genetics 2000). That organization subsequently defined genetic information as:

[I]nformation that derives directly from the variation between people that exists in their chromosomes or DNA, or information that is being used to infer that a specific genetic variation or genetic influences might be present. The former includes cytogenetic and DNA test results and very specific biochemical changes, whilst the latter category of genetic information includes family history, clinical diagnosis, imaging, clinical chemistry test results, etc. (European Society of Human Genetics 2000)

It is interesting to compare this broad definition with the more restrictive definition of what constitutes genetic testing given by the insurance industry. For example, the Investment and Financial Services of Australasia (IFSA) defines it for the purpose of its policy on genetic testing and insurance as "the direct analysis of DNA, RNA, genes or chromosomes for the purposes of determining inherited predisposition to a particular disease or group of disease but excluding DNA, RNA, gene or chromosome tests for acquired disease" (IFSA 1999). The Life Office Association of South Africa (2001), Association of British Insurers (ABI 1997) and Irish Insurance Federation (2001) have a similar view of what should be considered as a genetic test. The ABI (2001) also points out that "[W]hile there may be little or no conceptual distinction between molecular genetic information and other forms of predictive healthcare data, the popular perception appears to be that there is an important difference." The ABI differentiates between the impact of information resulting from molecular genetic testing and that from family pedigree information. The Canadian Institute of Actuaries (2000) goes further by stating: "[a] genetic test is a test to determine the presence or absence of particular variations in a person's genetic code." In short, "[d]istinctions between genetic and non-genetic information can be difficult to sustain, since most medical information can in one sense be considered genetic" (McGlennan 2000).

Yet, by distinguishing information coming from genetic tests from other genetic information or even other health information, guidelines of the insurance industry narrow the protection against genetic discrimination of an applicant. Insurers would probably argue, however, that if all genetic data were to be included within a given prohibition, the guidelines would become too general and unworkable (Lemmens 2000). Among their major concerns is the fact that a broad definition of genetic testing undermines currently accepted underwriting tools. Finally, any definition written into law today will most likely be applied to the next wave of demand for extending the prohibitions to long-term care insurance or for disability income insurance (Baker 2002).

In our overview of comparative positions in Europe, Australasia, and Asia, we discern five avenues that could or already do constrain access by life insurers to genetic information. The first is a human rights approach found mainly at international and regional levels. It includes an overriding prohibition on discrimination based on genetic characteristics or features. Within this approach, one can also include that of the Human Genome Organization (HUGO) Ethics Committee (1998), which recommended a broader interpretation of prohibited discrimination based on personal health data.

The second approach is found largely at regional and national levels. It limits the use of genetic testing or genetic test results to health care or research purposes. Outside of those therapeutic purposes, it forbids any other use of such information. A good example of this can be found in the 1992 European Convention on Human Rights and Biomedicine (1992) which states: "Tests which are predictive of genetic diseases or which serve either to identify the subject as a carrier of a gene responsible for a disease or to detect a genetic predisposition or susceptibility to a disease may be performed only for health purposes or for scientific research linked to health purposes, and subject to appropriate genetic counseling."

The third avenue requires that insurers be prohibited by law from performing genetic tests or inquiring about results of previously performed tests as a precondition for concluding or modifying an insurance contract. This approach is popular at international, regional, and national levels. Estonian legislation provides a good illustration, stipulating that: "Insurers are prohibited from collecting genetic data on insured persons or persons applying for insurance cover and from requiring insured persons or persons applying for insurance cover to provide tissue samples or descriptions of DNA" (Estonia 2001). An important distinction must be made among different instruments favoring prohibition in that some allow the insurer to have access to the applicant's genetic information with full informed consent, whereas others will not allow any access by the insurer even with consent of the applicant.

The fourth approach involves moratoria in which limitations on the use of genetic information for life insurance purposes come from the initiative of insurers themselves, although sometimes with government support. The strength of moratoria varies greatly from one country to another. Some insurers limit themselves to agreeing not to require genetic testing of applicants, whereas in other countries the results of previous tests will not be demanded. Some insurance moratoria have a ceiling over which it no longer applies; others apply to genetic information derived from research but not to clinical genetic test results.

A fifth approach is the status quo. The decision is not to legislate and to let the insurance industry decide what would constitute relevant genetic information for life insurance underwriting. All these approaches have strengths and weaknesses. Indeed, ultimately, the question is that of the responsibility of insurers as corporate citizens in modern societies where a universal health care infrastructure exists. Table 8.1 summarizes the laws of various countries.

The Human Rights Approach

UNESCO's Universal Declaration on the Human Genome and Human Rights states, "No one shall be subjected to discrimination based on genetic characteristics ..." (UNESCO 1997, article 6). By embodying the general antidiscrimination principle but extending the traditional list of

Table 8.1
Restrictions on the Use of Genetic Information by Insurers for Life Insurance Underwriting (as of August 2003)

Country	Moratorium[a]	Legislation[b]	Guidelines[c]	Convention on Human Rights and Biomedicine[d]	Other
Austria	No	Yes	No		
Australia	Partial	No	Yes		A bill on genetic privacy was introduced in 1998 but has not been accepted
Belgium	No	Yes	No		
Bulgaria	No	?	?	Ratified the Oviedo Convention 8/1/03	
Canada	Partial	No	Yes		
Chile	No	No	Yes		
Cyprus	No	No	No	Ratified the Oviedo Convention 7/1/02	
Czech Republic	No	No	No	Ratified the Oviedo Convention 10/1/01	
Denmark	No	Yes	Yes	Ratified the Oviedo Convention 12/1/99	
Estonia	No	Yes	No	Ratified the Oviedo Convention 6/1/02	
Finland	Yes, unlimited amount Exp: none	No	Yes		

Country					
France	Yes, unlimited amount Exp: 2004	Yes	Yes		A parliamentary commission declared that insurers should not use genetic test results
Germany	Yes, limited amount Exp: 2006	No	Yes		
Georgia	No	Yes	No	Ratified the Oviedo Convention 3/1/01	
Greece	Partial	No	Yes	Ratified the Oviedo Convention 12/1/99	
Hungary	No	No	Yes	Ratified the Oviedo Convention 5/1/02	
Iceland	No	No	No		A bill has been presented but has not been enacted
India	No	No	Yes		
Ireland	Yes, limited amount, some conditions excluded Exp: 2005	No	No		
Israël	No	Yes	No		
Italy	No	No	Yes		Guidelines for genetic testing to be adopted shortly by Ministry of Health
Japan	No	No	Yes		Association of Life Insurance Medicine has code of practice in preparation
Luxembourg	No	Yes	Yes		

Table 8.1 (continued)

Country	Moratorium[a]	Legislation[b]	Guidelines[c]	Convention on Human Rights and Biomedicine[d]	Other
Moldova	No	No	No	Ratified the Oviedo Convention 11/26/02	
Netherlands	No	Yes	Yes		
New Zealand	Partial	No	Yes		
Norway	No	Yes	Yes		
Portugal	No	No	Yes	Ratified the Oviedo Convention 8/13/01	Task force established by the Ministry of Health has prepared key guidelines addressing genetic testing
Romania	No	No	No	Ratified the Oviedo Convention 8/1/01	
San Marino	No	No	No	Ratified the Oviedo Convention 12/1/99	
Singapore	No	No	Yes		
Slovakia	No	Yes	No	Ratified the Oviedo Convention 12/1/99	
Slovenia	No	No	No	Ratified the Oviedo Convention 12/1/99	Bill should be drawn up shortly specifically addressing human genetics
South Africa	Partial	No	Yes		

				Bill prohibiting discrimination in insurance and employment has been presented
South Korea	No	No	No	
Spain	No	No	No	Ratified the Oviedo Convention 1/1/00
Sweden	Yes, limited amount Exp: Dec 2004	No	Yes	
Switzerland	No	Yes	Yes	
Turkey	Yes	No	No	
United Kingdom	Yes, limited amount, some conditions excluded Exp: 2006	No	Yes	

Source: Table prepared by Yann Joly.

Notes:

[a] Partial: the insurer will not ask the applicant to undergo genetic testing but may request results of genetic tests already taken by the applicant.

Ceiling: the insurer will not ask the applicant to undergo genetic testing or request results of genetic tests already taken by the applicant unless the insurance policy asked for is over a given amount.

Unlimited: the insurer will never ask the applicant to undergo genetic testing or request results of genetic tests already taken by the applicant.

[b] This category covers any legal protection restricting access to genetic information by insurers.

[c] This category covers any guidelines made by scientific or professional organizations regarding the restriction on the use of genetic information.

[d] States that have ratified this Convention are bound by it. The Convention forbids any kind of discrimination against a person based on genetic heritage. Genetic testing should be permitted only for health or research purposes.

prohibited grounds to include genetic characteristics, UNESCO considers such characteristics to be as inherent to the person as gender, age, and race. This approach is extended to personal data when it stipulates that: "Genetic data associated with an identifiable person and stored or processed for the purposes of research or any other purpose must be held confidential in the conditions set by law" (UNESCO 1997, article 7). It being in the very nature of a declaration to be proclamatory, it remains for other more binding instruments to reiterate such principles and to foresee their application with appropriate sanctions at the regional or national level. Nevertheless, the terms "genetic characteristics" and "genetic data" are telling in that they underscore the concept that the notions of mental or physical handicap and privacy of personal data are not sufficiently robust to include genetic information.

It bears noting that at the regional level, the Council of the European Union mirrored UNESCO's approach in prohibiting discrimination based on genetic features (Council of European Union 2000). Similarly, the Council of Europe's Convention for the Protection of Human Rights and Dignity of the Human Being with Regard to the Application of Biology and Medicine prohibits discrimination on grounds of genetic heritage (Council of Europe 1997a).

Prohibition against genetic discrimination and the need to preserve the confidentiality of genetic data and ensure their protection from access by insurers has received support from several international professional bodies (International Huntington Association 1994; Human Genetics Society of Australasia 1999). This approach is undermined, however, because life insurance is seen as a private contract sanctioned under national laws covering risk assessment and selection, subject only to the marketplace or to rules of professional practice and thus exempt from the general prohibition.

The HUGO Ethics Committee offers a variant in that it explicitly considers genetic information to be "like other medical information" and requiring human rights protection as such. This is consistent with the Council of Europe's Recommendation on the Protection of Medical Data, which includes genetic data in the concept of medical data (Council of Europe 1997b). The European Group on Ethics in Science and New Technologies of the European Commission (1999) also limits itself to stating that as concerns insurers "[s]uch third parties must in no case have direct access to personal health data." As mentioned, however, most countries do not consider it discriminatory to inquire about a person's health condition in the private contract of life insurance underwriting. In fact, as seen under the principle of mutuality, if prohibited from doing so, insurers would not be able to classify risk and the system would collapse. Thus, if health information is relevant and exists and the applicant is aware of it, it will have to be communicated.

The Therapeutic Approach

The Council of Europe's 1997 Convention for the Protection of Human Rights and Dignity of the Human Being with Regard to the Application of Biology and Medicine simply states that any genetic test "may be performed only for health purposes" (article 12), thereby thwarting specific requests by insurers for testing. The confidentiality of data is included under the general "right to private life in relation to information about his or her health" (Council of Europe 1997a, article 10).

The Convention on the Human Rights and Biomedicine has been ratified by a number of European countries. Indeed, Cyprus, the Czech Republic, Denmark, Estonia, Georgia, Greece, Hungary, Lithuania, Moldova, Portugal, Romania, San Marino, Slovakia, Slovenia, and Spain have agreed not only that genetic testing can be performed only for health purposes or for scientific research linked to health purposes, but also that any form of discrimination based on genetic heritage is prohibited. The Convention came into force in January 2000 after having been ratified by five states. Ratification procedures differ in each country, but normally involve parliamentary approval. Before ratification each state has to bring its laws into line with the Convention. This may require no change, a change to domestic legislation, or new laws. Domestic laws must include legal sanctions and require compensation for individuals who have suffered undue harm after medical treatment or research. As mentioned, genetic tests solely for insurance purposes or for exclusion solely on the basis of genetic heritage would be prohibited. Georgia, for example, made its internal legislation conform to the convention by including its restrictions concerning genetic material in a new Law on Patients Rights (Georgia 2000). It is interesting to note that even though neither Norway nor France ratified the Convention, both include in their legislation a prohibition on the study of the genetic characteristics of a person in the absence of medical or research purposes, thus mirroring the therapeutic approach of the Convention.

In Asia, this approach has also been recommended. In 1999, the Japanese Society for Familial Tumors (JSFT) presented draft guidelines stating that: "research should only be performed for the advancement of diagnostic, therapeutic and prophylactic procedures, as well as the understanding of the etiology and pathogenesis of the disease" (Kimura 1999). It also added that "the right to have access to genetic information belongs to the participant" and that "[t]he maintenance and confidentiality of genetic information should be strictly controlled in order to protect the privacy of the participant." The guidelines also stipulate that insurance companies should not inquire about genetic data. The Council Committee of Ethics of the Japan Society of Human Genetics (2000) also produced guidelines stipulating that even where consent is obtained "the utmost care is needed so that this information is not used as a source of discrimination."

The Prohibitive Approach

The third approach, which specifically restricts by law requests for genetic testing or access to results by insurers as a condition for issuing a life insurance policy, seems to be the most comprehensive. International organizations and

[g]overnments favoring this approach recognize that even though predictive genetic testing is not yet widespread, significant quantities of genetic information are already held in data banks and could be sought by insurers. A potential difficulty faced by an individual who is asked to consent to the disclosure of genetic information by an insurance company is that since the implications of such disclosure cannot be fully understood in advance, the consent given cannot be regarded as truly informed. (McGlennan 2000, p. 48)

Absent an explicit statutory prohibition on individual consent, this approach is somewhat limited in that if the individual consents, the private law of contracts governs it and the information cannot be withheld. Considering the latter, we saw that general legal obligations of disclosure by the applicant found in the law on insurance contracts would apply. Examples of such limitations can be found in the World Health Organization's 1998 Proposed International Guidelines on Ethical Issues in

Medical Genetics and Genetic Services, which state: "Genetic data should not be given out to insurance companies, employers, schools or governments, other than after the full informed consent of the person tested." The 1999 World Health Organization Statement on Cloning in Human Health reported that "[i]ndividuals have the right to retain control over their genetic material and the information derived from it. Access and use must be defined through consent, contract or law. Genetic information should not be used as the basis for refusing employment or insurance. Exceptions would have to be legally defined." Thus, only a statutory prohibition mentioning that individual consent is not an exception avoids the consent issue or the specific contractual rules of insurance.

It is interesting to note that on the regional level, the European Council Health Committee (1999) added a nuance to the concept of a total prohibition under law. The report stated, "[i]n order to take into account the legitimate interest of the insurer, who in all fairness, wishes to reduce the risk of adverse selection, it would be foreseeable to apply an exception to the non-disclosure of previous genetic test results to the insurers if the coverage desired is much higher than the financial status of the applicant" (p. 20). This proportionate approach is equitable in that it fulfills mutuality while avoiding adverse selection.

The prohibitive approach is particularly popular among European countries. Austria, Belgium, Denmark, Estonia, France, Luxembourg, The Netherlands, Slovakia, Sweden, and Switzerland have enacted laws specifically restricting access to genetic information. Except for Switzerland, the prohibition is total and cannot be set aside by consent of the applicant or rules of insurance law. In short, in most countries, prohibitive protection cannot be lifted even with individual consent. Outside of Europe, Georgia and Israel are the only countries that have legislated to prohibit insurers access to genetic information. In Asia, the Indian Council of Medical Research, without clearly indicating whether specific legislation is necessary, supports the prohibitive approach.

The Moratorium Approach

Insurers in several countries decided to state publicly that they will neither request life insurance applicants to undergo genetic testing nor divulge results of genetic tests previously undertaken.

The attractions of this strategy for the insurance industry are apparent. From the perspective of public relations, it enables the insurance industry to appear sensitive to public concern and responsive to criticism. This option has also a prestige enhancing effect for an industry in so far as it reflects a strong sense of moral responsibility on the part of the industry in question. In reality, it may well be the case that the current round of moratoria does not represent such a major concession to public opinion given that there are very few actuarially relevant and accurate genetic tests available. (McGlennan and Wiesing 2000, p. 374)

Insurance associations of Australia, Canada, Finland, France, Germany, Greece, Ireland, New Zealand, South Africa, Sweden, Turkey, and the United Kingdom have all adopted some form of moratorium. It can be self-regulated or a collaboration between major insurance associations and the government, as is the case in the United Kingdom and Sweden.

A derivative in the approach that is popular among several countries is a partial moratorium initiated by the industry. Major actuarial organizations of Australia, Canada, Greece, New Zealand, and South Africa have all stated their opposition to mandatory genetic testing for insurance. Yet they consider it acceptable to access existing test results of an applicant after obtaining consent. The IFSA claims that it will nevertheless "take account of the benefits of special medical monitoring, early medical treatment, compliance with treatment and the likelihood of successful medical treatment when assessing overall risk" (1999). Most associations also give the applicant, or the doctor, reasons for any adjustment made on insurance premiums related to the result of a genetic test.

Although insurers' associations of most countries that have moratoria agree that insurers should not demand that an applicant take a genetic test in order to obtain insurance, only in Finland, France, Germany, Ireland, Sweden, and the United Kingdom have insurers made a stronger commitment. These associations agreed not to ask an applicant for results of previous genetic tests but limit their engagement in various ways. A popular technique is for insurers to provide a time limit of usually no more than five years to the moratorium. This allows them to take some time to understand fully the process of underwriting or to renew the moratorium.

Another interesting feature of this approach is the possibility of a ceiling. Underscoring any intervention by government or insurers in Europe is the recognition that both social security and universal health care are in place. As mentioned, life insurance, while seen as a necessary socioeconomic good in modern society, is still a private contract subject to general rules. Thus, where the amount of life or disability insurance asked for exceeds a certain amount, results of genetic tests have to be supplied. The ceiling serves to distinguish the function of life insurance from social, state-sponsored schemes that are compulsory and based on solidarity as opposed to mutuality. Furthermore, a ceiling has long been a more general feature of medical testing and life insurance. It reduces the potential effects of adverse selection by permitting the insured to transfer risk only within narrowly constrained boundaries. It is assumed that the risk of adverse selection only truly comes into play with large amounts of capital. Individuals who know they are at higher risk might take out high-value policies that would have to be funded by other policy holders. This means that adverse selection can still occur within such a ceiling system, but actuarial models suggest that consequent increases in premiums would be negligible. For applicants, it permits acquisition of social goods such as cars and housing. Finally, a ceiling can also be proportionate to personal income levels as opposed to a set amount.

As concerns the combination of moratoria with government approval, the United Kingdom is illustrative. In 1997, the Association of British Insurers produced a code of practice in which not only were insurers barred from requesting genetic tests or requiring disclosure, but underwriters were not allowed to take into account what they knew about a given family. The subsequent creation of the Genetics and Insurance Committee had as its purpose the evaluation of tests proposed by insurers. Even though ultimately the committee considered that the test for Huntington disease is reliable and actuarially relevant, the controversy was such that the government imposed a further five-year moratorium on the use of genetic tests for insurance. In short, whereas the committee decision was accurate, the public was not ready for such transparency. We say transparency because it is obvious that insurers will obtain the same information by legitimate examination of family histories. Indeed, if one comes from a family with a history of this disease, one has a 50% chance of developing it, a factor that will be considered by insurers in any event and is known by family members. If one has the disease, like all the other medical conditions that are expressed, this will be taken into account. Thus, paradoxically, the true advantage of genetic testing would be to prove that one is risk free so as not automatically to pay the high premium. This moratorium gives the insurance industry the time to gather sufficient data. Even more salutary, it does not have the untoward effect of discouraging citizens from participating in genetic research or from testing. In any event, contrary to popular perception, other than in the case of monogenic conditions, research results are rarely of sufficient clinical significance (U.K. Forum 2001). The advent of predictive testing for genetic risk factors such as breast cancer tests for women, only make this time interval all the more important.

This condition-by-condition approval within a general moratorium agreed to by government together with the industry can be called reflective. This means that use of genetic tests in insurance is subject to oversight by government advisory bodies. It constitutes a policy option that mitigates the problems generally associated with genetics and insurance. In fact, the issue of actuarial relevance has become central to the debate on the topic. The position taken by the insurance industry (e.g., ABI in the U.K.) is that genetic test results will, in certain circumstances, be actuarially relevant. Moreover, if such information is useful to the applicant, it can also be useful to insurers. Insurers maintain that there is no difference between genetic information and other forms of data to which they have established access. Genetic information is one additional factor to be evaluated. In an area of rapidly developing technology, such a reflective system can react to changing circumstances. It implies that rational, scientifically sound, and empirically supported discrimination is permissible, as is the case under general antidiscrimination legislation.

The Status Quo Approach

As seen earlier, the life insurance system is based on mutuality. Insurers have to be able to rate risk appropriately to avoid the possibility of adverse selection. It could be maintained then, that insurers are best suited to decide whether a genetic test is sufficiently accurate or if a genetic condition is sufficiently serious to warrant mandatory disclosure. After all, they are on the edge of technologies that improve the latest diagnostic tools leading to discoveries (for example, implications of hypertension and obesity on mortality). Some of the most qualified experts in the fields of genetics work for insurance companies. Should it be up to the insurance industry to decide what is or is not actuarially relevant?

This approach seems to predominate in Asia. Japan and China have well-developed genetic testing technologies, and nothing restricts insurers from using resultant information. In this region, the dilemma has not yet aroused intense reactions by either governments or industry seen in Europe. In Singapore and Korea, the potential danger of imposing genetic testing before obtaining life insurance was brought up by several professional groups, but little legislative action has taken place. Several Asian countries have access to public health care, but life insurance in many of these countries is considered a luxury rather than a necessity.

It should be noted that the Japanese life insurance industry has shown increasing interest in genetic information. In a survey of companies, over half revealed they would like to adopt genetic testing of potential policy holders (Takagi 2000). Controversy surfaced, however, when children screened positive for two genetic disorders (Folling disease and phenylketonuria) were denied coverage, prompting protests from the Japanese Medical Association, which claimed the ban had no medical basis.

Conclusion

Taking the approaches in turn, there is no doubt that, at this time, the human rights approach when applied to the arena of life insurance is limited in its potential and may unwittingly encourage discrimination. The terms "genetic characteristics" and "genetic data" are telling in that they underscore the fact that the notions of mental or physical handicap or of the privacy of personal or medical data under current legislation are not sufficiently robust to include genetic information. Indeed, we contend that singling out genetic features or data can only exacerbate the perceived abnormality of genetic conditions or at-risk status, thereby contributing to further stigmatization and discrimination. General antidiscrimination legislation also fails to address the fact that fair insurance practices usually constitute an exception to such legislation. Insurance is seen as a private contract sanctioned by law as a risk-assessment business subject only to the marketplace or rules of professional practice.

The therapeutic approach at a minimum avoids the pitfalls of the human rights approach by addressing the purpose of testing rather than singling out genetics and so draws a much wider net. In fact, prohibition on genetic testing outside of therapeutic purpose would allow the inclusion of social attributes within the prohibition, as would mere perception of being at risk for a genetic condition. We mean that unless considered scientifically validated, such tests would not be performed for insurance purposes nor would mere perception of at-risk status be sufficient. Thus, tests for social attributes such as agression would be precluded. Nevertheless, the value of the therapeutic approach is also limited in that the results of persons participating in genetic research are not adequately protected, the status of research records being uncertain. Furthermore, once a test is performed, its result would have to be communicated if requested by the insurer. This not only affects individual participation but also the request of another family member for pedigree or linkage analysis since familial data are shared by underwriters. Obviously, the legitimate and traditional use of family history questionnaires also thwarts this approach.

In contrast, explicit legislative prohibitions have the sociopolitical allure of the quick fix but in fact may be overreaching, because even persons from at-risk families or in the general population who test negative cannot profit from their health status. Furthermore, the time is near when genetic testing will include testing for proteins, for gene-drug interactions, and for gene-environment exposure. What then constitutes a genetic test or information? Is it possible to distinguish between the results of these tests and family history questionnaires? Moreover, the line between genetic and medical information is necessarily blurred as genetic factors increasingly appear in common diseases as opposed to single-gene conditions. The latter development also obscures the confidentiality of genetic, medical, or personal data through the protection offered by notions of personal privacy or medical confidentiality.

The moratorium approach offers a diversity of techniques that can be adapted to different cultures and legal systems. It can also include agreements between industry and the government, thereby adding political weight and oversight. Yet, not all countries have a single insurance payer or consortium of life insurers so the extent of coverage may be narrow, to say nothing of the issue of monitoring insurers to see what occurs in actual practice. Furthermore, will the time frame be used for actively validating and updating actuarial tables in this age of genetic complexity and of little knowledge of the role of environmental factors? Such a time frame should also be used to study the consequences of possible access to genetic testing results. Actuarial fairness is the cornerstone for legitimate discrimination.

We maintain that in the moratorium approach, the system of a set ceiling amount with appropriate levels of minimum coverage for all, or of a ceiling proportionate to level of income replacement value, limits the risk to industry of adverse selection. At best, this may be the most realistic, albeit temporary solution.

Finally, the status quo approach (in other words, bide your time and ride it out) rests on dual assumptions that competitive forces in the market will prevent undue discrimination and that insurers are not currently using or asking for genetic test results. The latter is borne out in the literature, which is beginning to illustrate the absence of actual genetic discrimination in insurance practices. In fact, studies reveal that alleged discrimination by applicants was often based on misunderstanding of normal insurance practices or of genetic information and of the nature of genetic disorders (Wertz 1998–1999). In the same vein, even when those affected with a genetic disorder applied for insurance, the fear of insurers that people would buy an excessive amount of insurance (adverse selection) did not materialize either (Hall and Rich 2000; Barlow-Stewart 2000).

Obviously, misunderstanding and allegations by both sides of the debate argue for more than the continuation of the status quo. Most important, they illustrate that public perception and insurer misgivings require the same form of intervention. What then, should be done?

We suggest both a moratorium, preferably under a ceiling or proportionate approach, in concert with governmental approval through an oversight body. Such a body can constantly update, publish, and integrate scientifically validated information, and through public participation regain not only public trust but also public understanding of the workings of the industry. The positive aspects of genetic testing also must be considered, for example, medical surveillance, early treatment, and its likelihood of success.

More important, we also argue in favor of the adoption of legislation that is not genetic specific. The first possible avenue is to add to human rights legislation that prohibits discrimination based on sex, race, and physical or mental handicap the phrase "or the perception thereof." This would explicitly include within the purview of the general list of prohibitions at-risk but asymptomatic persons, who often are perceived as being already affected. It would also include social attributes often mistakenly attributed to familial genes.

The second avenue is to reinforce legislated protection of medical data and research data generally. In this way, it is hoped that individuals and families will not fear genetic testing or participation in research since all medical data will be better protected. Access by third parties should be strictly limited by law to certain defined situations and questions (i.e., no fishing expeditions). All medical data, including genetic data, will thereby receive greater protection.

Finally, it goes without saying that exclusion from life insurance remains a *real* risk in the absence of a compulsory and comprehensive health care system based on solidarity. This third avenue is the cornerstone.

It is our hope that by these three avenues, current fears based on perceptions of genetic abnormalities and of the socioeconomic impact on insurance will not further exacerbate stigmatization and discrimination. Indeed, with integration of genetics into more general legislation, it could serve as a tool for larger social and political change. The normalization and integration of genetic information depends on it.

References

Anderlik, M. R. and Rothstein, M. A., "Privacy and Confidentiality of Genetic Information: What Rules for the New Science?" Annu. Rev. Genomics Hum. Genet. 2: 401–433 (2001).

Association of British Insurers, Genetic Testing Code of Practice, www.geneticinsuranceforum.org.uk/Code/menu.asp (1997).

Association of British Insurers, Insurance and Genetic Information, www.abi.org.uk/ResearchInfo/InsuranceandGeneticInfo (1997).

Baker, C. D., "When Genetic Testing Collides with Major Medical Insurance," Contingencies, March/April 2002, pp. 35–36.

Barlow-Stewart, K., "Genetic Discrimination in Australia," J. Law Med. 8: 251 (2000).

Canadian Institute of Actuaries, Statement on Genetic Testing and Insurance, www.actuaries.ca/publications/2000/20065f.pdf (2000).

Council of Europe, Convention for the Protection of Human Rights and Dignity of the Human Being with Regard to the Application of Biology and Medicine: Convention on Human Rights and Biomedicine, article 11, Int. Digest Health Legis. 48: 1, 99, (1997a).

Council of Europe, Recommendation no. R (97) 5 of the Committee of Ministers to Member States on the Protection of Medical Data, http://cm.int/ta/rec/1997/97r5.html (1997b).

Council of the European Union, Charter of Fundamental Rights of the European Union, www1.umn.edu/humanrts/instree/europeanunion2.html (2000).

Estonia, Human Gene Research Act, article 27(1) (2001).

European Committee of Insurance, Medical Examinations Preceding Employment or Private Insurance, www.cea.assur.org/cea/v1.1/posi/uk/frame04.msql?position_id=12 (1998).

European Council Health Committee, The Medical Examination for a Contract of Employment and/or Private Insurance: Proposal of Direct European Lines, http://www.coe.int/T/E/Social_Cohesion/Health/Documentation/Medical%%examinations%%PUB%%English.asp (1999).

European Group on Ethics in Science and New Technologies (EGE), Opinion no. 13, Ethical Issues of Healthcare in the Information Society, http://europa.eu.int/comm/European_group_ethics/docs/avis13_en.pdf (1999).

European Society of Human Genetics, Genetic Information and Testing in Insurance and Employment: Technical, Social and Ethical Issues, www.eshg.org/insurance.htm (2000).

Georgia, Law on Patients' Rights (2000).

Hall, M. A. and Rich, S. S., "Genetic Privacy Laws and Patients' Fear of Genetic Discrimination by Health Insurers: The View From Genetic Counselors," J. Law Med. Ethics 28: 245 (2000).

Human Genetics Society of Australasia, Predictive Genetic Testing and Insurance, www.hgsa.com.au/policy/pgti.html (1999).

Human Genome Organization Ethics Committee, Statement on DNA Sampling: Control and Access, www.hugo-internation.org/hugo/sampling.html (1998).

International Huntington Association, Guidelines for the Molecular Genetics Predictive Test in Huntington's Disease, www.huntington-assoc.com/guide1.htm (1994).

Investment and Financial Services Association, IFSA Standard on Genetic Testing Policy, http://www.ifsa.com.au (2002).

Irish Insurance Federation, Code of Practice on Genetic Testing, www.iif.ie.codes.htm (2001).

Japan Society of Human Genetics, Council Committee of Ethics, Guidelines for Genetic Testing, www.medic.kumamoto-u.ac.jp/dept/pediat/jshg/jshg-kaikoku-3-5-Eng.htm (2000).

Kimura, R., "Genetic Diagnosis and Gene Therapy in the Cultural Context: Social and Bioethical Implications in Japan," in Gene Therapy and Ethics, Nordgren, A., ed. Stockholm: Elandes Gotab (1999).

Lemmens, T., "Selective Justice, Genetic Discrimination, and Insurance: Should We Single out Genes in Our Laws?" McGill Law J. 347 (2000).

Life Office Association of South Africa, Code of Conduct, Code on Genetic Testing, www.loa.co.za/codeofconduct/Chapter21 (2001).

McGlennan, T., "Legal and Policy Issues in Genetics and Insurance," Commun. Genet. 3: 45 (2000).

McGleenan, T. and Wiesing, U., "Insurance and Genetics: European Union Policy Options," Eur. J. Health Law 7: 367 (2000).

Read, A., "Genetics and Insurance," Genet. Law Monit. 2: 4 (2002).

Takagi, S., "Genetic Counseling Sadly Lags Behind Technology," Asahi Shimbun May 25 (2000).

U.K. Forum for Genetics and Insurance, Association of British Insurers, and British Society for Human Genetics, Joint Statement on Genetics and Insurance, announced at the Royal Society, April 24, http://www.ukfgi.org.uk%20 statement%20abi%20bshg,%20ukfgi%2024%2004%2001.htm (2001).

UNESCO, Universal Declaration on Human Genome and Human Rights, www.unesco.org/human_rights/hrbc.htm (1997).

Wertz, D. C., "Genetic Discrimination: Results of a Survey of Genetics Professionals, Primary Care Physicians, Patients and Public," Health Law Rev. 7: 3–7 (1998–1999).

World Health Organization, Proposed International Guidelines on Ethical Issues in Medical Genetics and Genetic Services, http://wwwlive.who.ch/ncd/hgn/hgnethic.htm (1998).

World Health Organization, Cloning in Human Health, http://www.who.int/wha-1998/WHA99/PDF99/ew12.pdf (1999).

9

Antitrust Implications of Insurers' Collaborative Standard Setting

Robert H. Jerry II

Whenever two or more market participants collaborate to restrain trade, the potential applicability of federal and state antitrust laws must be considered. When the collaborating parties are insurance companies, a further layer of analysis may be necessary to determine whether the activity is exempt from federal antitrust regulation. Even if the activity enjoys an exemption under federal law, state antitrust law may have different things to say about the activity. Embedded in each of these levels of analysis are many difficult and complex subsidiary questions. In short, the law of insurance antitrust is not a subject for the faint of heart.

Insurers collaborate in many situations. They have long cooperated in drafting standard policy forms, sharing data regarding the identification and quantification of risks, and collecting and disseminating loss and expense data. They also have a long tradition of cooperating in setting rates in the fire and casualty lines. For the most part, these collaborative activities are exempt from federal antitrust scrutiny by the McCarran–Ferguson Act, and similar exemptions at the state level to the application of state antitrust laws also protect these practices. Yet very few industry precedents exist for collaborative insurer agreement or standard setting with respect to the use or nonuse of particular underwriting criteria in setting the terms of insurance coverage or the price charged for it (or both). The absence of such examples is not surprising. If a particular underwriting factor is actuarially unsound, no compact is required to discourage insurers from using it. If the factor is actuarially sound, insurers will be loath to surrender their ability to use it, and no advantage is to be accrued from arranging a compact among insurers pursuant to which all agree to use the factor.

It is possible to imagine, however, circumstances in which insurers might perceive the formation of such a compact to be advantageous. For example, with respect to whether they should surrender their option to use genetic information in life insurance underwriting, a seemingly reasonable, innocuous suggestion might be made: life insurers should voluntarily agree to place a moratorium on using genetic information in underwriting. With little current use of such information, now might be the time to forge such an agreement. The collaboration is appealing from egalitarian and distributive justice perspectives, but antitrust law has implications in situations where its relevance is least expected, as many who have credentials as antitrust offenders know well. Such a moratorium is essentially an agreement among competing insurers to fix one determinant of the product's price, and this restraint of trade calls into question the possible applicability of federal and state antitrust law (as well as the relevance of possible exemptions under federal or state law, or both). Several antitrust issues would accompany the articulation and implementation of such a moratorium or other agreement related to genetic information.

Federal Antitrust Laws and Anticompetitive Insurer Conduct

The federal antitrust statute with the most relevance to the insurance industry is the Sherman Act, the substance of which rests in two brief but sweeping provisions enacted by Congress in 1890 (15 U.S.C. §1 et seq.). Section 1 is the "restraint of trade" provision; it is relevant to many kinds of collaborative conduct, including horizontal restraints among competitors. Section 1 states: "Every contract, combination ... or conspiracy, in restraint of trade or commerce among the several States, or with foreign nations, is ... illegal." Section 2, the "monopoly abuse" provision, states: "Every person who shall monopolize, or attempt to monopolize, or combine or conspire with any other person or persons, to monopolize any part of the trade or commerce among the several States, or with foreign nations, shall be deemed guilty of a felony...." The presence of monopoly power (classically defined as the power to control prices or exclude competition) is not enough to make out a violation of section 2; rather, the offender must possess monopoly power plus engage in anticompetitive conduct to obtain, use, or preserve it.

Because most insurance markets do not have a single insurer with dominant market power, section 2 has less practical importance to the insurance industry than section 1 (Insurance Antitrust Handbook 1995). Nevertheless, section 1 is the provision relevant to concerted insurer conduct to eliminate use of one or more underwriting factors when determining coverage or premium levels.

The statutory language of the Sherman Act depends on judicial interpretation and construction for its content. As the U.S. Supreme Court stated in *Apex Hosiery Co. v. Leader* (1940), "[t]he prohibitions of the Sherman Act were not stated in terms of precision or of crystal clarity and the Act itself did not define them. In consequence of the vagueness of its language ... the courts have been left to give content to the statute." But in doing so, courts must adhere to the Act's purpose: "The Sherman Act was designed to be a comprehensive charter of economic liberty aimed at preserving free and unfettered competition as the rule of trade.... [T]he policy unequivocally laid down by the Act is competition" (*Northern Pacific Railway Co. v. United States* 1958).

Whether challenged insurer activity violates federal antitrust law is a question that, at least in theory, is preliminary to whether the insurer activity enjoys an exemption from federal antitrust law. Although the analysis necessary to determine the applicability of an exemption can be very complicated, sometimes deciding the exemption question is easier than determining whether the challenged conduct is an antitrust violation. Thus, it can be expedient to proceed initially to the exemption analysis rather than grapple with the question of antitrust liability. The following discussion, however, visits the antitrust liability issue first and then proceeds to the exemptions.

The text of section 1 begins with the phrase "contract, combination ... or conspiracy." Each term requires cooperative conduct by at least two actors, that is, two (or more) sellers, two (or more) buyers, or a seller and buyer (or more) in combination (Shenefield and Stelzer 2001). In some circumstances, this concerted action requirement can be met by the activity of a trade association or similar group. The reference to "several States, or with foreign nations" means that the trade restrained by the concerted action must be either in or at least have an effect on interstate or foreign commerce; incidental commerce that is entirely intrastate in character and impact is not the concern of section 1. Because every contract restrains trade by obligating the contracting parties to deal only with each other with respect to the contract's subject matter, a literal reading of section 1 would invalidate all contracts, an obviously untenable result. In 1911, the U.S. Supreme Court, drawing on the common law of unfair competition, interpreted section 1 as prohibiting only *unreasonable* restraints of trade (*Standard Oil Co. of N.J. v. United States* 1911), and this reading has been reiterated on numerous occasions.

The meaning of "unreasonable restraint" evolved along two lines. First, "there are certain agreements or practices which, because of their pernicious effect on competition and lack of any redeeming virtue, are conclusively presumed to be unreasonable" (*Northern Pacific Railway Co. v. United States* 1958, p. 5). These kinds of restraints, such as direct price fixing, bid rigging, division of markets among competitors, some kinds of boycotts (i.e., concerted refusals by competitors to deal with third parties), and resale price maintenance, are deemed to be unreasonable per se. The logic of this categorization is that courts have determined from experience that some kinds of restraints are so fundamentally anticompetitive and so lacking in justification that no analysis beyond the determination of the fact of their existence is necessary to determining invalidity.

The second line of analysis is known as the "rule of reason." With respect to any activity not per se unreasonable, relevant circumstances must be evaluated to determine whether the conduct is, on balance, procompetitive or anticompetitive. The rule of reason is the prevailing standard under section 1 of the Sherman Act. For example, a bona fide joint venture (to be distinguished from a sham joint venture, which is a subterfuge for an agreement to fix prices and is therefore unreasonable per se) may be a legitimate effort to achieve efficiencies that promote, rather than stifle, competition (Insurance Antitrust Handbook 1995, pp. 13–14). Most vertical agreements (agreements between companies at different levels of product distribution, such as a manufacturer and wholesaler), as distinct from horizontal agreements (agreements among competitors), are tested under the rule of reason (ABA Section of Antitrust Law 1997, pp. 73–74). Although an agreement to fix one or more components of price may be a per se violation, "courts have applied the rule of reason rather than the per se rule where ... the relationship between the restraint and price is sufficiently attenuated" (ABA Section of Antitrust Law 1997, p. 77). Social considerations are generally excluded from rule of reason analysis: "Because the rule of reason focuses on the restraint's competitive effect, factors unrelated to competition—with possible rare exceptions for health and safety considerations and for deviations from the traditional profit-maximizing business model such as the professions, municipalities, and universities—are generally irrelevant" (ABA Section of Antitrust Law 1997, p. 54).

Courts have generally "declared unlawful per se agreements among competitors to raise, lower, stabilize, or otherwise set or determine prices" (ABA Section of Antitrust Law 1997, p. 77). Price fixing is not limited to setting the ultimate price. Credit terms, trade-in allowances, cash down-payment requirements, discounts, free service, or any other element of price that is the subject of competitor agreement can constitute a per se unlawful restraint. Other less direct connections between the activity and price, such as agreements to use specific accounting methods, to require a percentage contribution from each contract to an industry-wide collective bargaining fund, or to use only particular subcontractors, are also deemed per se violations of section 1 (ABA Section of Antitrust Law 1997, pp. 81–82). Agreements to "fix some element of price or the process by which price is determined ... do not fix the price as such, [but] they do require participants to compute the price in a certain way.... Once such an agreement is appropriately classified as naked, per se condemnation follows as a matter of course" (Hovenkamp 1999).

Allegations of concerted action are not always based on alleged formal agreements among competitors. Frequently, they are based on patterns of uniform business conduct, which is commonly referred to as "conscious parallelism." The presence of legitimate business reasons that would lead firms independently to follow the same course of action or the absence of motive for a conspiracy exemplify the kinds of considerations that will rebut the allegation of conscious parallelism. Because insurers tend to compete rather than cooperate with respect to risk classification determinations, it is improbable that a conscious parallelism argument would succeed with respect to such determinations. Thus, if antitrust claims are to have viability, it will be with respect to demonstrated, formal collaborations among insurers.

In insurance, the product is the insurance policy, and the price of the product is the premium. If insurers agree among themselves to fix the level of premiums, they are engaged in price fixing in violation of the Sherman Act; unless the anticompetitive conduct earns an antitrust exemption, the insurer combination constitutes a per se violation of section 1. Similarly, when two or more insurers agree that a particular underwriting factor will not be used in determining the level of premiums, they are taking a factor relevant to the ultimate cost to the consumer and agreeing to eliminate this factor as a basis for competition. In other words, when insurers surrender the right to make price distinctions based on a particular underwriting factor, they forfeit the ability to segregate a risk class and offer members of subdivided classes a differentiated product based on coverage or price (or both). All of this has the effect of stabilizing price in the relevant market by eliminating competition based on a component of product price. This, too, falls within the category of restraints that courts traditionally deem per se violations of section 1.

As noted above, if the relationship between the restraint on a component of price and the ultimate price is sufficiently attenuated, courts have applied the rule of reason rather than the per se rule in assessing the restraint. If insurers agree not to use a particular underwriting factor in determining premiums, it is arguable that the impact on price is more attenuated in that competition can still occur with respect to other underwriting factors, thereby diluting the impact on price of the agreement. This does not validate the restraint, but does provide a basis for testing it—and possibly upholding it—under the rule of reason.

If the rule of reason is the appropriate standard for testing a restraint's validity, the question becomes whether the restraint "is one that promotes competition or one that suppresses competition" (*National Society of Professional Engineers v. United States* 1978, p. 691). Exactly how this analysis would play out in the case of insurer agreements involving underwriting criteria is difficult to predict. On the one hand, competition would be enhanced because consumers whose genetic profiles indicate higher risk would have access to insurance that would otherwise not be available at all or would be available only at higher rates. But consumers whose genetic profiles do not indicate higher risk or that affirmatively demonstrate lower risk would not be able to receive the advantages of their genetic profiles. When these consumers are grouped with consumers whose risks are higher, competition is impaired.

In the same vein, consumers whose family history puts them in a higher-risk group would not be able to use genetic information to negate assumptions normally drawn from adverse family history; for them, competition is reduced. It is by no means obvious that the procompetitive virtues of a restraint on use of genetic information in underwriting outweigh the anticompetitive aspects; thus, it cannot be assumed that the restraint would pass muster under the rule of reason.

Because a restraint on the use of genetic information furthers egalitarian values and public policies that encourage equal treatment of individuals based on factors beyond their control, the question arises as to whether these justifications count in the restraint's favor under a rule of reason analysis. As noted earlier, social considerations are generally excluded from rule of reason analysis. For example, in *National Society of Professional Engineers v. United States* (1978), the U.S. Supreme Court rejected the professional organization's argument that a provision in its canon of ethics prohibiting competitive bidding by members was necessary to prevent inferior engineering work and to protect the public's health, welfare, and safety. The Court reasoned that its role was "not to decide whether a policy favoring competition is in the public interest, or in the interest of the members of an industry" (p. 692) because the Sherman Act reflects Congress's judgment that competition "will produce not only lower prices, but also better goods and services," and that under the rule of reason inquiry into "the question of whether competition is good or bad" (p. 675) is not permitted.

The restraint in *Professional Engineers* is arguably distinguishable from an insurer-imposed restraint on use of an underwriting factor in that the professional association's restraint on competitive bidding is directly beneficial to the economic self-interest of the association's members, whereas the insurance restraint does not eliminate competitive bidding but merely alters the terms on which insurers' competition for business occurs. If a constraint on the use of genetic information in underwriting has any economic benefit for insurers, it is highly indirect and much less significant to the insurers than the restraint in *Professional Engineers* was to the parties imposing them.

The economic self-interest factor was important to the Third Circuit's analysis in *United States v. Brown University*, in which an agreement among universities on financial aid to be offered students to eliminate a bidding war among the universities for top applicants was at issue (*United States v. Brown University* 1993). The universities maintained that the agreements were designed to help make more money available for needy students, and the district court rejected this justification as an inappropriate social, noneconomic justification. The Third Circuit disagreed, reasoning that the aims of the financial aid agreement would increase the quality of the educational product by increasing socioeconomic diversity on campuses, and would increase consumer choice by making high-quality education available to more students, unlike the restraint in *Professional Engineers*, which reduced consumer choice. The Third Circuit remanded the case to the district court for full rule of reason analysis.

How the choice-enhancing factor that aided the restraint in *Brown University* plays out in the insurance context is difficult to assess. On the one hand, it might be contended that a restraint on the use of genetic information in underwriting increases consumer choice by making insurance available to more persons. Those who would have been denied insurance or offered it only on limited terms due to negative genetic information are benefited if insurers cannot take such information into consideration. On the other hand, applicants who do not have negative genetic information would presumably be rated as lower-risk insureds and would have access to lower-cost insurance if insurers did not foreclose their ability to make underwriting distinctions based on genetic information. How these two factors would be balanced by a court, and whether, ultimately, the restraint would be determined to achieve a net procompetitive effect, is difficult to predict.

Perhaps a more likely outcome is that courts would observe that prohibiting life insurer use of genetic information in underwriting is something that the legislatures could do; after all, many state legislatures have taken precisely that position with respect to health insurance, and a few have done so with respect to life insurance. Failure of some legislatures to include life insurance in statutes prohibiting use of genetic information in health insurance underwriting stands as an indirect but deliberate statement of policy that such a prohibition is not desired, at least at this time. In some states, the relevant statute has an explicit carve-out for life insurance. In circumstances where legislatures decline to elevate egalitarian values with respect to the use of genetic information in life insurance underwriting, a court may decline to take it upon itself to elevate such values.

Courts have also interpreted section 1 as placing limitations on competitors' ability to agree not to deal with, or to deal only on particular terms with, other entities. These arrangements are typically described as "group boycotts" or "concerted refusals to deal." Early cases treated these combinations as per se violations of section 1, but more recent cases tend to analyze such restraints under the rule of reason. Exactly how one draws the line between a refusal to deal that is per se unlawful and one that receives rule of reason treatment is difficult to articulate.

In the insurance context, the argument might be made that an agreement among insurers to deal with individual applicants only on terms that make no distinction based on genetic information constitutes a boycott or concerted refusal to deal. Authority for this position comes from cases such as *Sandy River Nursing Care v. Aetna Casualty* (1993), where the First Circuit held that concerted efforts by insurers to refuse to offer certain types of insurance coverage in an attempt to induce the Maine legislature to authorize rate increases was "an economic boycott that beyond doubt 'constituted a classic restraint of trade within the meaning of Section 1 of the Sherman Act'" (p. 1143) and was per se unlawful. (The boycott was ultimately exempted from the antitrust laws by virtue of the state action doctrine, which is discussed below.) Although this kind of concerted conduct is unlawful under the Sherman Act, the antitrust exemption provided by the McCarran–Ferguson Act immunizes it.

Industry self-regulation efforts can also give rise to allegations of concerted refusal to deal. One of the most common examples involves industry enforcement of trade association membership criteria. If, for example, an association member deviates from association guidelines, other members might take steps to sanction the offender, perhaps through actions that exclude the offender from markets. Industry associations sometimes also set standards for product quality or safety, occasionally offering certifications for products that meet the standards. When a particular firm's product is excluded from or disadvantaged in the market on account of its failure to meet such standards, the firm might claim that the association's standards constituted an unlawful restraint on trade. When challenged, such standards are usually evaluated under the rule of reason: "Key factors determining whether ... standard-setting or certification programs restrain trade are the extent of the economic detriment they cause to an excluded or nonqualifying firm, the breadth of restrictions in relation to their need, and how the standards are used. In considering the manner in which standards are used, courts have considered whether the application of nominally acceptable rules is designed to suppress competition" (ABA Section on Antitrust Law 1997, pp. 112–113).

Product standard setting is common in the insurance industry; most notable is the practice in many lines of insurance of creating standard forms. When challenged, courts noted the procompetitive aspects of this practice in that standardization makes it easier for consumers to compare prices of alternative products. If insurers were to agree that policy pricing would not be based on certain criteria, it could be contended that this combination constituted the equivalent of a trade association standard or perhaps standardization of the product itself. Those who could claim disadvantage from the practice would be consumers who would have benefited if the underwriting criterion had been used (in this context, consumers lacking genetic characteristics that would have been disadvantageous in the underwriting process), and perhaps firms that wish to market policies based on genetic distinctions if efforts to exclude these firms from the market accompanied promulgation of the standard. Evaluation of the standard would proceed under the rule of reason, and it is difficult to predict what conclusions courts would draw when applying the rule.

The McCarran–Ferguson Federal Antitrust Exemption

Although the McCarran–Ferguson Act is often described as a statute preempting federal antitrust law, it does much more than that. Its most important purpose is to give primacy to state regulation of the insurance business to the extent that states choose to regulate the industry, at least to the extent that Congress opts not to reassert its primacy, as it can at any time or in any specific context. Yet because the Act's emergence can be traced to the concern of stock fire and casualty companies about the application of antitrust laws to their business, its antitrust implications are significant.

The Supreme Court held that insurance transactions were subject to federal regulation under the Commerce Clause (*United States v. South-Eastern Underwriters Association* 1944). This also meant that the insurance industry was subject to federal antitrust statutes. In response, the industry and the National Association of Insurance Commissioners rallied behind federal legislation to limit the impact of the decision. One year later, the result was the McCarran–Ferguson Act (15 U.S.C. §§1011–1015).

The substantive core of the McCarran–Ferguson Act is contained in section 2:

(a) The business of insurance, and every person engaged therein, shall be subject to the laws of the several States which relate to the regulation or taxation of such business.

(b) No Act of Congress shall be construed to invalidate, impair, or supersede any law enacted by any State for the purpose of regulating the business of insurance … unless such Act specifically relates to the business of insurance: *Provided*, That after June 30, 1948, [the Sherman Act, the Clayton Act, and the Federal Trade Commission Act] shall be applicable to the business of insurance to the extent that such business is not regulated by State law.

Section 2(a) states that the "business of insurance" (a phrase not defined in the Act) is appropriately within the domain of state regulation. The portion of section 2(b) before the proviso functions as a reverse preemption statute; Congress uses its commerce power to state that no act of Congress will preempt state law unless Congress is explicit that it intends such preemption to occur. Because antitrust laws are general statutes that do not "specifically relate" to insurance, they would be applied to the insurance business if the text of section 2(b) ended before the proviso, but the section 2(b) proviso creates a limited antitrust exception. The proviso does not explain what kind or intensity of regulation is necessary to trigger the exemption. Furthermore, section 3(b) created an exception to the section 2(b) antitrust exemption by stating that the Sherman Act applies to some insurer activities regardless of what regulation the states might enact: "Nothing contained in this chapter shall render the said Sherman Act inapplicable to any agreement to boycott, coerce, or intimidate, or act of boycott, coercion, or intimidation." None of the three practices listed in section 3(b) is defined in the statute.

When the meaning of the McCarran–Ferguson Act for antitrust enforcement is digested from its provisions, the following formula emerges: if a federal antitrust law is sought to be applied to an insurer activity, the activity—(1) if it constitutes the business of insurance—is exempt from such regulation (2) to the extent that such business is regulated by state law and (3) the challenged insurer activity does not constitute a boycott, coercion, or intimidation.

For many years after McCarran–Ferguson was enacted, it was widely assumed that federal antitrust law—and state antitrust law as well—had limited relevance to the activities of insurance companies. However, two U.S. Supreme Court decisions—*Group Life and Health Insurance Co. v. Royal Drug Co.* in 1979 and *Union Labor Life Insurance Co. v. Pireno* in 1982—construed the Act narrowly, thereby exposing insurance companies to increased antitrust scrutiny. This narrowing of immunity has continued during the past twenty years, perhaps reflecting a view that immunity was initially construed too broadly, or perhaps that it has become unnecessary in light of the availability of the state action immunity (Areeda and Hovencamp 2000, pp. 322–323).

In applying the McCarran–Ferguson Act, the threshold question is whether the challenged insurer activity involves the business of insurance. If this question is answered in the negative, the insurer conduct enjoys no protection from antitrust analysis. Under the *Royal Drug–Pireno* test, three questions are asked in determining whether an insurer's activity constitutes the business of insurance: does the activity involve the underwriting or spreading of risk? does the activity involve an integral part of the insurer-insured relationship? and is the activity limited to entities within the insurance industry? None of the three factors is necessarily determinative.

To satisfy the first element, the insurer's activity must have "the effect of transferring or spreading a policyholder's risk" (*Union Labor Life Insurance Co. v. Pireno* 1982, p. 129). Transactions in which the insurer does not assume risk and distribute it across a pool of similarly situated insureds in similar transactions will not meet this test. If, for example, the insurance product is primarily an investment, such as variable life insurance or a variable annuity, it may not involve the spreading of risk and thus may not be the business of insurance. The second part of the *Royal Drug–Pireno* test was derived from *Securities and Exchange Commission v. National Securities, Inc.*, where the Supreme Court stated that section 2(b) was designed to protect from impairment, invalidation, or preemption by congressional action state laws concerned with the relationship between the insurance company and its policy holders (*Securities and Exchange Commission v. Variable Annuity Life Insurance Co. of America* 1959). If the insurer's activity has only an indirect effect on the reliability of the insurer or on the insurer-insured relationship, that minimal effect is not enough to qualify the activity as the business of insurance. To satisfy the third part of the test, it is necessary to show that the challenged insurer activity is limited to entities within the industry.

Under the three-part test, it is well settled that rate-making activity constitutes the business of insurance for purposes of the McCarran–Ferguson Act. Scope of coverage, including the content of policy provisions, is very closely connected to rate making; thus, joint activities with respect to scope of coverage also fit within the business of insurance. Although joint insurer conduct with respect to underwriting criteria has not been directly challenged or the subject of a judicial decision, such agreements also are likely to fall within that ambit. Consequently, an agreement by life insurers not to use genetic information as an underwriting factor would rest at the core of the business of insurance.

When the statute sought to be applied to an insurer's activity is a federal antitrust law, the analysis becomes more complicated because of the section 2(b) proviso, which requires that the insurer activity be regulated by state law to prevent application of federal law. The difficulty with this language is its ambiguity with respect to what kind of regulation is necessary and the extent to which it must be effective to avoid the regulation of federal antitrust law. In applying this language, courts have been disposed to treat statutes of general applicability, such as corporation codes, general business and professional codes, and state antitrust laws, as laws that regulate the business of insurance.

Is concerted insurer activity with respect to the use of underwriting criteria, and with respect to criteria on the use of genetic information in particular, regulated by state law? No state statute gives explicit approval to such restrictions. As discussed in chapter 11, at least forty-five states regulate some aspect of genetic testing in health insurance, and many of these statutes restrict insurers' underwriting practices. A few states extend these prohibitions to life insurance underwriting. The fact that legislatures in many states opted not to regulate underwriting in life insurance at the same time they enacted such regulations in health insurance suggests that the states made a judgment about the extent to which regulation of underwriting with respect to genetic information should occur.

In addition, unfair trade practice statutes of most states contain unfair discrimination prohibitions that specifically reference sex, marital status, race, religion, and national origin. The omission of genetic characteristics (other than sex and race) from this list could be viewed as a deliberate legislative assumption that insurers should not be subject to regulation with respect to their use of information relevant to such characteristics. Unfair trade practice statutes have generally not been held to prohibit underwriting criteria that are actuarially fair, and sex and marital status often figure prominently in underwriting in some lines of insurance in many states (Meyer 1993). Although one might contend that this demonstrates that the use of genetic information in underwriting is not regulated by state law, courts' disposition to treat statutes of general applicability as the kinds of laws that regulate the business of insurance strongly suggests that the unfair trade practices statutes are specific enough to satisfy the regulated by state law requirement. This supports the proposition that insurer underwriting practices with respect to genetic information do enjoy an antitrust exemption.

The territoriality question could serve in some situations to limit the scope of the exemption. Assuming insurer activity that operates and has its impact nationally, effective regulation of the activity in state A does not provide an exemption for the activity's operation and impact in state B; only if state B also regulates the activity does it enjoy the benefit of an exemption in state B. All states have unfair trade practice regulations, but not all have genetic information underwriting regulations. To the extent the exemption's existence depends on genetic information regulation, it is possible that a national business practice could enjoy the exemption in some states but not in others.

Finally, if one seeks to subject an insurer's activity to Sherman Act scrutiny, section 3(b) of the McCarran–Ferguson Act states that the Sherman Act will apply even if the insurer's activity constitutes the business of insurance, and even if state law regulates it, if the activity involves a boycott, coercion, or intimidation. Based on the Supreme Court's narrow construction of the term "boycott" in *Hartford Fire Insurance Co. v. California* (1993), it is clear that if insurers agree to use particular underwriting criteria and do not use this agreement to try to extract favorable terms from third parties on collateral transactions, a section 3(b) boycott is not involved and the exception to the antitrust exemption is not triggered.

Based on the Supreme Court's narrow construction of the term "boycott," it is clear that if insurers agree to use particular underwriting criteria and do not use this agreement to try to extract favorable terms from third parties on collateral transactions, a section 3(b) boycott is not involved and the exception to the antitrust exemption is not triggered.

State Action Exemption, or Parker Doctrine

Under the state action doctrine, restraints of trade that are the product of state regulatory policy are exempt from the antitrust laws. Sometimes called the *Parker* doctrine after the U.S. Supreme Court decision that is its cornerstone (*Parker v. Brown* 1943), antitrust immunity is given to private parties as long as their conduct is authorized and regulated by the state. It is not enough for the state to immunize private conduct that would otherwise be unlawful, as would be the case if the state simply authorized private actors to fix prices; rather, the state must be involved so that the competitive restraints constitute "state action or official action directed by a state" (*Parker v. Brown* 1943, p. 351).

The test for determining the availability of the exemption has two elements: "First, the challenged restraint must be 'one clearly articulated and affirmatively expressed as state policy'; second, the policy must be 'actively supervised' by the State itself" (*California Retail Liquor Dealers Association v. Medical Aluminum, Inc.* 1980). The clear articulation prong is met if the state clearly intends through the enactment of a regulatory scheme to displace competition in a particular market. Specific detailed legislative authorization of the restraint of trade is not required, and it is only necessary that the statute permit, as opposed to require, the anticompetitive conduct. The active supervision prong is met if state regulators have the statutory authority to review the challenged anticompetitive conduct and actually exercise that authority.

Exactly how vigorous state review must be to create state action immunity is uncertain. *In Federal Trade Commission v. Ticor Title Co.* (1992), the Supreme Court found the active supervision test was not met where statutory review authority over rate filings existed, and the insurance department was "staffed and funded" and showed "some basic level of activity" in enforcing the rating law. (*Federal Trade Commission v. Ticor Title Co.* 1992). Thus more aggressive state regulation is required to create *Parker* immunity than is necessary for McCarran–Ferguson Act immunity, but existing case law does not quantify this difference. The difference between the two regimes is largely academic, as it is difficult to imagine a situation in which the *Parker* doctrine would confer immunity in circumstances when insurer activity is insufficiently regulated by state law to obtain McCarran–Ferguson immunity (Kintner and Bauer 1989, p. 249).

Nevertheless, in those few states that presently limit life insurers' use of genetic information in underwriting, an agreement among insurers not to use such information would be immune from antitrust liability under the *Parker* doctrine. Whatever anticompetitive impact would arise from such a restraint would be absolutely irrelevant under antitrust law by virtue of the doctrine. Also, if similar statutes were to be adopted in other states, insurers in those states would be absolutely immune from antitrust liability. As noted above, many states have statutes that prohibit the use of genetic information in the underwriting of health insurance policies. These statutes should not be viewed as constituting state action that immunizes collaborative conduct by life insurers with respect to that information. Enactment of a health insurance regulation does not carry a clearly stated legislative purpose to authorize the anticompetitive conduct in life insurance and does not put in place state mechanisms that supervise private conduct in this area.

In other words, the state action doctrine does not immunize life insurers from antitrust liability for joint agreements to forego using genetic information in underwriting, except in states where the use of such information is prohibited by state statute. The fact remains, however, that by exercising their prerogative to regulate and supervise insurers' use of genetic information in life insurance, the states could create federal antitrust immunity under the state action doctrine. If a few states enacted such legislation and life insurers, acting independently, conformed their underwriting practices to the requirements of these states, this conduct should not be deemed an unlawful combination triggering antitrust scrutiny.

The related *Noerr–Pennington* doctrine, named for two U.S. Supreme Court decisions that articulate the doctrine's substantive core, gives antitrust immunity to restraints that derive from legislative, regulatory, or judicial decisions resulting from joint lobbying or litigation efforts of competitors (*Eastern Railroad Presidents Conference v. Noerr Motor Freight, Inc.* 1961; *United Mine Workers of America v. Pennington* 1965). The protected conduct is the petitioning of the government to restrict competition in the marketplace. Standard setting by a private association is not protected by this doctrine; rather, the restraint must flow from government action. Thus, life insurers would be free to collaborate to petition state legislatures to adopt statutes that would eliminate underwriting based on genetic factors, but *Noerr–Pennington* would not protect an agreement among life insurers to stop using that information in underwriting.

Under existing authority, it is doubtful that joint insurer lobbying of the National Association of Insurance Commissioners (NAIC) would be protected by the *Noerr–Pennington* exemption, even though the NAIC is a voluntary body of government regulators. Because *Noerr–Pennington* immunity is grounded in a First Amendment right to petition the government, the fact that the NAIC is not a government entity, even though its membership consists of government officials, means that collaboration to lobby the NAIC would test the limits of *Noerr–Pennington* immunity.

State Antitrust Laws and Anticompetitive Insurer Conduct

Generally speaking, state antitrust laws use language that tracks closely the federal statutes, and state courts give federal cases varying degrees of precedential value, but there are notable deviations from both propositions. According to one compilation, forty-eight of the fifty states have general antitrust statutes, and twelve states have statutory provisions specifically exempting some insurance-related activities (Insurance Antitrust Handbook 1995, pp. 34–36). Several states have statutes that incorporate federal exemptions, most notably the McCarran–Ferguson exemption and the state action doctrine, into state law. But many states have no such exemption and some generally refuse to find any immunity for insurance companies from state antitrust law. Twenty-one states have a generic exemption for regulated industries, including insurers; these exemptions are usually functional equivalents of the state action doctrine (Insurance Antitrust Handbook 1995, pp. 36–37). It is difficult to generalize about state exemptions, except to say that in many states they are limited.

About a decade ago, state antitrust law became more significant for the insurance industry. State enforcement became more aggressive and more coordinated, and some states repealed part or all of the provisions giving state antitrust immunities to the insurance industry (Insurance Antitrust Handbook 1995, p. 33). In 1988, California voters approved Proposition 103, which repealed the insurance antitrust exemption and substituted two safe harbors limited to the exchange of certain historical data and participation in state-approved residual market mechanisms. Thereafter, the legislature restored an exemption for joint development of standard policies. In 1990, New Jersey eliminated its exemption for joint ratemaking in the private passenger automobile insurance market except for "collection, compilation and dissemination of historical data." In 1991, Texas eliminated its exemption based on McCarran–Ferguson and substituted an exemption for "actions required or affirmatively approved by any statute of this state ... or by a regulatory agency of this state." Since this flurry of activity a little over a decade ago, state legislatures appear to have given relatively little attention to insurance antitrust issues.

It is impossible to summarize here the antitrust law of the fifty states, but as a general proposition, insurers cannot be assured without careful study of the law of individual states that they will enjoy the same breadth of immunity from antitrust enforcement in the states as they do at the federal level. As a result, insurers will be reticent to engage in collaborative conduct, particularly if the perceived benefits from the conduct are relatively limited.

Conclusion: The Impact of Uncertainty

Although insurers are in the business of assuming and distributing risk, they are risk averse, just like the individuals and firms who pay premiums to transfer risk to them. Risk-averse actors assign probabilities to outcomes of conduct, and if expected benefits of an activity do not exceed expected losses, the activity will not occur.

As a matter of antitrust law, there is no impediment to individual life insurers unilaterally rejecting the use of genetic information in underwriting. The Sherman Act and its state counterparts subject collaborative behavior between two or more market participants to antitrust scrutiny, not unilateral conduct. But individual insurers are not likely to renounce the right to use this information. As long as genetic information is thought to have the potential to help insurers make more precise risk classifications and more accurately price coverage, no insurer is likely unilaterally to subject itself to the comparative disadvantage that goes with renouncing a viable, or potentially viable, rating tool. If genetic information has predictive power for risk classification, the insurer that ceases to make distinctions based on the information will attract higher-risk insureds to its pools. The insurer that uses the information to make distinctions will be able to offer lower-risk insureds a more favorably priced product. This in turn will cause lower-risk insureds to depart the pool of the insurer that declines to make such distinctions. Ultimately, that insurer will be forced to raise premiums to cover its higher-risk pool, which in turn will drive more insureds out of the pool. Left uncorrected, this adverse selection spiral will result in collapse of the pool. The only circumstances in which an insurer should seriously contemplate unilaterally surrendering an underwriting tool is if the insurer is convinced that other insurers will follow suit. But in a competitive market, the insurer should anticipate that some other insurers will decline to do so in order to gain the comparative advantages that accompany the use of an underwriting tool with predictive power.

If unilateral surrender is not viable, the question becomes whether concerted action by several insurers could achieve the same result. For the same reasons discussed above, it is unlikely that insurers would be able to forge an industry-wide moratorium on the use of genetic information because of the industry's inability to police the moratorium effectively against nonconforming insurers. The possibility of competitive advantage from violating the moratorium means that the moratorium would not be accepted on an industry-wide basis. In these circumstances, some insurers might endorse the moratorium in principle but would be unwilling to subscribe to it knowing that complete adherence is impossible.

Moreover, even if such an agreement could be reached, collaborative conduct would raise the antitrust issues discussed above. Collaborative insurer standard setting with respect to use of genetic information in underwriting would probably pass muster under the federal antitrust laws (provided the policies involved are insurance products, as opposed to financial investment devices that do not involve spreading and distributing risk). Greater uncertainty exists under state laws, particularly for insurers whose business is multistate. Because the costs of being wrong about the lawfulness of such conduct are so significant, the conclusion that joint conduct is *probably* lawful is insufficient to cause insurers to proceed with the activity. A prominent insurance treatise explains the problem in this way:

The pervasive uncertainty about how antitrust principles will be applied in different insurance contexts chills not only the ardor of the more aggressive competitors but also the willingness of many insurers to participate in collective mechanisms to serve various public policy objectives. The threat of litigation is real. Antitrust law permits, even encourages, such actions by providing for treble damages.... The possibility of treble damages, the creativity of plaintiff antitrust lawyers, the potential of large and hugely expensive class action litigation, the civil and criminal penalties available to the government, and the uncertain results when applying antitrust law to insurance all tend to stifle even activity that might ultimately pass antitrust muster. (Hanson 2000)

Only if collaborative conduct promises benefits more substantial than the risks associated with possible antitrust liability would the rational insurer be interested in joining the agreement. The cost-benefit calculus does not favor concerted action to surrender a viable underwriting tool.

The creation of an explicit statutory immunity for collaborative insurer activity with respect to underwriting factors, or with respect to the use of genetic information in particular, would remove antitrust uncertainty, but it would not alter competitive forces that make a multi-insurer agreement unlikely in the first place. As is often the case, industry movement to a particular underwriting standard occurs only if the movement is universally adopted, which will not occur absent compulsion by some external authority (such as government regulation). Thus, the most effective way to achieve a moratorium or any regulation of insurers' use of genetic information in life insurance underwriting is to prohibit the practice outright, as many states have done with health insurance and some have done with life insurance. This, however, turns the discussion full circle to the fundamental question underlying the discussion in this book: whether it is feasible and desirable to prohibit life insurers from using genetic information in underwriting and, if so, whether such prohibitions are politically achievable in the legislative arena.

References

ABA Section of Antitrust Law, Antitrust Law Developments, vol. 1, Chicago: American Bar Association, 4th ed. J. Angland, ed. (1997).

Apex Hosiery Co. v. Leader, 310 U.S. 469 (1940).

Areeda, P. E. and Hovencamp, H., Antitrust Law, vol. 1, New York: Aspen Law & Business. 2nd ed. (2000).

California Retail Liquor Dealers Ass'n v. Midcal Aluminum, Inc., 445 U.S. 97, 105 (1980).

Eastern Railroad Presidents Conference v. Noerr Motor Freight, Inc., 365 U.S. 127 (1961).

Federal Trade Commission v. Ticor Title Ins. Co., 504 U.S. 621 (1992).

Group Life and Health Insurance Co. v. Royal Drug Co., 440 U.S. 205 (1979).

Hanson, J. S., "The Regulation of Life Insurance, Part 2," in McGill's Life Insurance, 3rd ed., E. E. Graves and L. Hayes, eds. New York: American College (2000).

Hartford Fire Insurance v. California, 509 U.S. 764 (1993).

Horning, M. F. et al., eds., Insurance Antitrust Handbook: A Project of the Insurance Industry Committee, Section of Antitrust Law. Chicago: American Bar Association (1995), p. 18.

Hovenkamp, H., Antitrust Law vol. 12, ¶ 2020. New York: Aspen Law & Business (1999).

Kintner, E. and Bauer, J. P., Federal Antitrust Law: A Treatise on the Antitrust Laws of the United States. Cincinnati: Anderson Publications (1998).

Meyer, R. B., "Justification for Permitting Life Insurers to Continue to Underwrite on the Basis of Genetic Information and Genetic Test Results," Suffolk University Law Rev. 27: 1271 (1993).

National Society of Professional Engineers v. United States, 435 U.S. 679 (1978).

Northern Pacific Railway Co. v. United States, 356 U.S. 1 (1958).

Parker v. Brown, 317 U.S. 341 (1943).

Sandy River Nursing Care v. Aetna Casualty, 985 F.2d 1138 (1st Cir.), cert. denied, 510 U.S. 818 (1993).

Securities and Exchange Commission v. Variable Annuity Life Insurance Co. of America, 359 U.S. 65 (1959).

Shenefield, J. H. and I. M. Stelzer, The Antitrust Laws: A Primer, 4th ed. Washington, DC: AEI (2001).

Standard Oil Co. of New Jersey v. United States, 221 U.S. 1 (1911).

Union Labor Life Insurance Co. v Pireno, 458 U.S. 119 (1982).

United Mine Workers of America v. Pennington, 381 U.S. 657 (1965).

United States v. Brown University, 5 F.3d 658 (3d Cir. 1993).

United States v. South-Eastern Underwriters Association, 322 U.S. 533 (1944).

10

A Consumer Agenda

J. Robert Hunter

Major Considerations From a Consumer Perspective

Genetic Advances Reopen a Fundamental Question: Is Insurance a Right?

We have, through Medicare, decided that health insurance is a right for seniors, and through Medicaid, determined the same for the poor. Several states have plans to cover uninsurables. We are currently engaged in debate about how the system will cover other health insurance uninsureds. One way or another, we have allowed people to gain access to health care through free clinics or otherwise; a sloppy system compared with national health plans of other nations, but a system nonetheless. Health insurance has emerged as a clear right as part of modern life in the entire developed world outside of the United States and a quasi right here.

Norman Daniels (2004) argues that moral considerations lead him to conclude that limits should be placed on the private market-driven system for health insurance because health insurance is a fundamentally important social good. The question of whether some level of life insurance, an economic necessity when certain conditions pertain in modern life (e.g., the desire to reproduce and care for the child that is born), should be viewed as a right has never been debated fully in America. The Human Genome Project has opened a debate, which is, at the root, about this much broader question: Has life insurance become a right in the modern world?

The answer to this question is not as clear in life insurance as it is in health insurance. In order to need health insurance the sole condition is being born. Everyone needs health insurance. This is not obvious when it comes to life insurance. With a dependent, such as when a couple becomes pregnant, one or both of the expectant parents then need life insurance. That baby-to-be has about two decades of absolute dependence ahead. It is quite normal that the first time a couple seriously considers life insurance is when they first become pregnant. From the consumer perspective, this is the right choice because most people do not really need life insurance before then, and consumer groups have so advised consumers for decades.

Single people without dependents do not need life insurance, nor does a child at birth. A senior, whose children are grown and who has properly prepared for retirement financially, does not need life insurance, because life insurance is designed to protect against adverse financial consequences of premature death. Yet, through illness or death of close family members, events can precipitously lead one of these people suddenly to have a dependent. Everyone is at some risk of needing such coverage sometime in life. Society has decided that we will care for a baby if it becomes orphaned, or if a single parent becomes destitute and has no relative or other caregiver who can care for the child. So we have a system in place for the eventuality of premature death or unexpected illness leaving a helpless life to maintain.

There is a moral issue pertaining to the availability of affordable life insurance coverage under certain conditions. Consider a hypothetical situation. A woman has become pregnant and she and her husband need life insurance. Should the life insurance industry be absolutely free to demand a genetic test in that situation even if the result might surprise the couple with news they did not know or have reason to anticipate? What happens when the couple finds out that their expected child cannot have the protection afforded by life insurance for the breadwinning parent, either due to underwriting-based rejection or by pricing beyond the couple's ability to afford coverage? Will the couple be able to continue that pregnancy? If their religious beliefs disallow termination of the pregnancy, will the child be forced into the possibility or likelihood that it will become a pauper and require the state to pay for what its parents were willing to arrange?

Just as at birth the newborn child creates an absolute need for health coverage, the infant also has an absolute future death ahead and a genetically built-in drive to reproduce; a drive some say is as strong as the survival instinct. Besides being born, obviously that child might find itself, sometime in its lifetime, with a dependent to care for from death or illness of family members.

So, whereas consumers are not so naïve as to believe that unlimited life insurance should always be available to all comers, and they understand the need for private life insurance companies to prosper and to avoid adverse selection, we believe that there is a moral obligation for some amount of life insurance to be available and affordable for those with dependents. It surely would be difficult and costly to have to prove who needs life insurance. For example, if a father has a stroke and requires family support, are all of his children eligible? Are the man's siblings also eligible? To overcome this obviously difficult determination, every American should be eligible for a minimum amount of life insurance at a standard rate.

It is also necessary to explore the issue of social acceptability of the use of the genome in life insurance underwriting and pricing. For many years, life insurers charged nonwhite persons more than white persons. That ended decades ago because the nation decided that race-based rates were wrong. Now, the nation must engage in the discussion of social acceptability of the use of genetic information to underwrite or price people out of the market.

The industry understands that life insurance may be a right in our society. One large insurer has gone well beyond the proposals made above. In 2002 MassMutual announced it will issue 40,000 ten-year term policies of $50,000 each free to low-income parents of dependents (primary provider and eligible for the federal earned income tax credit). The death benefit will be limited to children's education. They did this in recognition of the finding of the American Council of Life Insurance that only 18% of Americans living at or below the poverty line have any life insurance (MassMutual 2002).

History Tells Us to Enact Laws Before Insurers Use Genetics

Consumers understand how the system works to entrench industry practices, even bad ones. Once genetic testing starts to be used, the industry will vigorously defend its continued use much in the same way it is defending its use of credit scoring as a classification and underwriting tool in auto and home insurance. Currently, in about forty states, legislatures are seeking to prohibit or limit the use of such scores on behalf of consumers. Although insurance company advocates cannot explain why someone who is laid off for a few months and falls a bit behind on some bills becomes a poorer driver, the industry is resisting substantive controls on the use of such scores.

Furthermore, once some insurers start using a practice, it is inevitable that others will follow out of fear of being adversely selected against. Thus, although years ago Blue Cross/Blue Shield sought to retain community rating of individual health insurance, they had to relent and start using age, health, and other pricing criteria because their competitors were taking younger and healthier risks away from them. In a similar fashion, the use of genetic information will surely become universal once even one insurer starts to use it to gain a competitive advantage. The insurer that uses the most refinement in classification often sets the standard to which all others eventually migrate out of concern for adverse selection.

Competition promotes efficiency and technological progress, but it can have an adverse effect in insurance. An insurer can gain an advantage by not writing certain sections of town (red-lining) or by up-rating minorities in life insurance (race-based pricing), to give just two examples. Even after legal prohibition, examples of persistence in these practices exist that only legal actions by harmed persons have been able to weed out. Consumers have a vital stake in getting protection in place now, before insurers start using genetic tests and other genetic information.

Analysis of Policy Options from a Consumer Perspective

Current State of the Law

About one-third of states have enacted consumer protections against inappropriate use of genetic tests in underwriting and/or pricing of life insurance. The protections are typically prohibition on unfair genetic discrimination, a requirement that actuarial justification precede use of genetic information, and a requirement that genetic tests cannot be used without informed consent of the consumer (National Conference of State Legislators 2002).

Yet these laws do not protect consumers adequately. They do not address many concerns related to privacy, quality of tests, access to insurance at a reasonable price, and others. The laws rely on the industry's own definitions of actuarial soundness, which result in abuse in other contexts. There are typically no clearly defined enforcement measures, no private rights of action, and no penalties specified.

Furthermore, the industry seems to say that it cannot do things jointly to assure consumer protection since, it claims, it would run afoul of federal and state antitrust laws (Jerry 2004). The McCarran–Ferguson Act allows insurers to take joint actions if regulated by the state. Insurers could, if they so desired, work out controls on the use of genetic test results in life insurance, subject to state involvement and active oversight without fear of violating antitrust law. For them to say that they cannot act together, under state regulation, to agree on ways to control their use of this information, and then to turn around and say that they must adopt the use of such information once it is in the marketplace to avoid adverse selection, takes chutzpa.

General Principles

The discussion of applicable principles generally tracks the format of chapter 11.

Consumers subscribe to the following principles:

1. Do not discourage at-risk individuals from undergoing genetic testing.
2. Do not coerce individuals into undergoing genetic testing.
3. Do not promote harmful social consequences, including genetic reductionism, determinism, and fatalism.
4. Make life insurance coverage available at affordable rates to as many people as possible.
5. Anticipate likely scientific developments.

Consumers, however, have at least some concerns with the principle that life insurance policies should promote actuarially sound underwriting and assure the public that underwriting and pricing decisions are fair. Two factors must be in place before insurance companies can use genetic tests for underwriting or pricing: assurances that insurers using such factors fully understand the science and can explain it to consumers, and actuarial data showing that the impact on mortality of the genetic factor must be credible, reliable, and fully explained to consumers.

Consumers also question the degree to which policy development should be structured to avoid adverse selection. They understand that an insurer must protect itself from adverse selection. That means, if regulation does not control the use of genetic tests, the insurer that most aggressively uses such tests and most aggressively applies every scrap of results to deny coverage or price risks will ultimately establish the standard for all insurers. We have witnessed this race to segmentation in other lines of insurance, such as auto insurance, where territories have been segmented down to ZIP Codes, credit scores are used, and tier rates are set up to twelve tiers in an insurer.

This race to ultrarefinement in classification and risk assessment must be dealt with by controls now, before we start down the road toward great refinement in genetic classifications used by underwriters and actuaries. This does not mean that persons with knowledge of some adverse genetic situation should be allowed to purchase unlimited amounts of life insurance. It does mean that consumers want protection at least up to some amount of coverage, such as the $100,000 level as proposed later in this chapter.

Existing laws are woefully inadequate to protect consumers from abuse by the life insurance industry. One need only recall cases from the 1990s leading to huge lawsuits and payment by leading insurers of billions of dollars in restitution. The state regulatory system has not been repaired to the extent necessary to assure America that these abuses will not occur again (Consumer Federation of America 2000).

The industry is seeking even more freedom from regulation by proposing an optional federal charter system in which insurers could choose between a federal or state regulator. Insurers making such a proposal admit that they want to set up an optional system so that levels of government would compete with each other for insurers by lowering standards, setting up a "race to the bottom" in regulation. Consumers cannot trust the life insurance industry or state regulators to protect them fully from improper uses of genetic information. Only explicit laws with clear standards are acceptable, and then only if a private right of action to enforce such standards is part of the package.

Consumers think it is inappropriate for policy making to be based on not creating a regulatory system that is overly complex or costly. Until we know for sure what should be in place, how can we agree to a principle that the ultimate system cannot be complex or costly? This idea of anticipating the future development of these matters is at odds with the principle of anticipating scientific developments.

Aspects of regulation of the use of genetic information will be complex. The regulator must understand genetics to come up with lists of acceptable tests for insurers if that is an aspect of the system. If the science develops in certain ways, the regulatory system must keep pace and may, by the nature of the science, be complex and costly. This is particularly true if there is no safety net of a guaranteed layer of life insurance protection. Accordingly, the principle should be to minimize regulatory complexity and costs consistent with achieving required protections.

Finally, consumers do not believe that developing recommendations that are politically feasible should be a priority. If we limit ourselves to the politically feasible now, we will not give pure advice on what is right. The political process will determine feasibility. We should construct the best policies, regardless of what ones may eventually be adopted. To limit recommendations based on our understanding (or misunderstanding) of what can be obtained politically will result in public policies that are even less than what is politically feasible. If we start out bending to where the political pressures are (insurers), insurers will push further, and the ultimate compromise will be, by necessity, less than what was attainable if the starting point was simply what was right and moral to protect people from the industry's future use (and misuse) of genetic information.

Genetic Exceptionalism

From a consumer perspective, if we cannot control the use of genetic information because it is too difficult to separate this information from other medical information, this other medical information will also have to be controlled by regulation. This will give incentives to underwriters and actuaries to find ways to separate as much of this other information as possible. One way to divide it is to document what other medical information is in use today by life insurers and restrict expansion of the use of any new classifications without an approval process, in which consumers would have the opportunity of review and comment.

Whereas it may be difficult to make a moral case for exceptional treatment, the fact is that use of genetic information by insurers is emerging as a tool, but is not one yet. Thus, control of it, including an outright ban on it (except when the applicant has the information), is possible and does not put insurers in a worse position than the status quo. To the extent that a guaranteed layer of coverage is available at affordable prices, the need to control genetic information is reduced.

Procedural Reforms

The process surrounding the use of medical information must be fully transparent, regulated, and accountable. First, the genetic testing industry must be regulated if for no other reason than it is new and the accuracy of the tests has yet to be determined by proper study. Later, statistical analysis of historical evidence must be undertaken. The need for such research is illustrated by an in-depth study undertaken by consumer groups of financial histories of consumers. It revealed that credit scores are based on often-erroneous data and approximately 20% of the population may be charged inappropriate mortgage interest rates as a result (Consumer Federation of America 2002). The public must be assured that genetic tests are reliable.

Even if genetic information is accurate, the actuarial implications of a particular genetic outcome must also be accurate. Actuarial proof is different from genetic scientific proof. Both must be in place before life insurers use the information in underwriting or pricing. Thus, laws must be passed that require use only of approved tests. Consumers will not settle for a list of disapproved tests since the regulatory lag will mean that newly developed "bad" tests will affect them until regulators catch up with new testing approaches.

The National Association of Insurance Commissioners by itself should not be tasked with coming up with such a list. The commissioners are too close to the insurers (fully 50% of commissioners come from and 50% go back to insurance industry employment). They do not have expertise remotely able to do this work, and they are known for the incredibly slow pace of their deliberations. This job should be given to a scientific body people trust, such as the National Institutes of Health.

Part of the transparency should be making public all underwriting guidelines and pricing schemes of each insurer. Making these documents public would help assure that no insurer violated restrictions and would give consumers knowledge of which insurers would be best for them, improving shopping capability and focus, and thereby enhancing competition.

I believe it is necessary to regulate testing laboratories. I also support the regulation of medical decision makers. Consumers want genetic decisions, to the extent that they are allowed, to be made by persons competent to make them. If life insurers must employ board-certified specialist physicians to accomplish that, so be it. If that requires phasing in, in the interim the company should be restricted from using tests requiring specialist personnel.

Informed consent would be required for all medical examinations and tests. Furthermore, physicians should be liable for adverse consequences of errors made in these procedures. Consumers should also be told exactly the intent of how a proposed test would be used, what the underwriting guide is related to the test, pricing implications of the outcome, and how results will be maintained to assure privacy and protection for family and loved ones.

Life insurers should be required to disclose the medical basis of an adverse underwriting decision. In addition, consumers should have access to complete underwriting-pricing guidelines so that they can determine if the adverse action is proper.

Consumers also should have a right to appeal an adverse underwriting decision. They need strong rights, not just for information, but also for convenient and fast methods to redress improper decisions. Private rights of action to enforce proper treatment of consumers should accompany these rights.

Consumers fear their most personal information being used in objectionable ways. Insurers must agree to requirements that genetic information must not be given to others or used for anything other than the specific purpose to which the consumer agreed *in advance in writing*. In no case should this information be used across product lines or to underwrite family members. Consumers should have access to information held by the insurance company to make sure it is timely, accurate, and complete. They should be notified periodically how they can obtain such information and how to correct errors. Consumers should not be denied policies or services because they refuse to share information (unless the requested information is necessary to complete a transaction and regulatory approval has been obtained for such use generally). Consumers should have meaningful and timely notice of the company's privacy policy and their rights and how the company plans to use, collect, and/or disclose personal information. Insurance companies should have a clear, approved set of standards for maintaining the security of information and have methods to ensure compliance. Privacy protections should not be denied to beneficiaries and claimants because a policy is purchased by a commercial entity rather than by an individual.

Finally, to counter undue industry influence, an independent, national public insurance counsel or ombudsman with adequate funding is necessary. Consumers must be well represented for the process to be accountable and credible. This should include sufficient resources to assure representation before regulatory entities that is independent, competently and adequately staffed, external to regulatory structure, and empowered to represent consumers before both administrative and legislative bodies.

Substantive Options

The critical issue for consumers is the need for substantive control of genetic information. Government must impose such controls on life insurers as soon as possible since the longer we wait, the stronger (and more vehement) will be insurers' insistence that limits on use of genetic tests will seriously affect their business practices or standards. In other lines of insurance, attempts to restrict methods sometimes result in letters to insureds, frightening them into believing that any change will have dire consequences for their rate or even availability of a policy.

As indicated at the outset of this chapter, consumers believe that there is moral equivalence with the concept that health insurance is a right when certain conditions obtain at the request to purchase life insurance. I do not see life insurance as merely a commercial transaction, a product to be allowed to flow freely in the competitive marketplace without interference by regulation. Solvency regulations and guarantee associations have been imposed for decades in this nation, since dependents relying on the proceeds of a life insurance policy cannot be abandoned when the named insured dies.

The idea of a right of access to some level of insurance has not been clearly debated in the United States. Consideration of moratoria, as well as other substantive and procedural control proposals in the context of the debate, make it clear that the subject of a right to life insurance is ripe for discussion. A solution such as establishing a maximum amount of coverage that could be bought without genetic tests is an example of this debate.

Life insurance, up to a certain amount, such as $100,000, should be a right when a person has a dependent (be it a by birth, marriage, adoption, or death or injury making a relative dependent on the proposed insured). Because of the complexity of defining all of the possibilities of when a person might have a dependent (if a parent is ill and must be cared for, is it all children who should have the right to obtain coverage, or grandchildren, or other close relatives, or all of the above?), I call for all Americans to be given a one-time right to a minimum level of life insurance protection (say $100,000, indexed for inflation) at standard rates.

Several European countries have adopted moratoria on the use of genetic information for medical underwriting in life insurance, including France, Germany, and the United Kingdom (Knoppers et al. 2004). Rothstein (2004) considers moratoria as "declaring the desirability of 'genetic free' underwriting ... the equivalent of legislation banning genetic testing and/or the use of genetic information." This may turn out to be true, but it is speculation. I am unsure if that would be the effect of such a moratorium, but this option should not be dismissed out of hand.

Another option is to prohibit genetic testing and using genetic information. Consumers believe that, if the debate about the moral need for all Americans to have a guaranteed layer of life insurance results in such a program, the price should not be based on health information, genetic or otherwise. This would obliterate the need to differentiate between genetic and other health information, and we would have no unequal protection issues to worry about.

A third option is to prohibit insurers from requiring genetic testing, but permit the use of the information. The concern that people might cheat and hide information regarding genetic tests and thus be in a position to select adversely against an insurer is no different than the concern that an applicant is hiding health information. Insurers routinely handle the latter through questions on the application and physical examinations, coupled with a right to rescind, ab initio, a policy obtained fraudulently or through material misrepresentation.

I envision that physical examinations, questionnaires, and testing as well as all other free-market means would be available to insurers for levels of insurance in excess of the guaranteed layer of coverage. The availability of guaranteed, no test, no physical examination coverage would minimize the need for testing, and the negative consequence of testing should not be as serious a deterrent for at-risk people when a test is appropriate. Since this proposal would not require tests, disclosure of medical information, or other tests, there would be no different treatment of genetic and other tests.

The idea I support as the way to deal with life insurance in the new world of genetics is to establish a maximum amount of coverage that can be obtained without genetic testing or genetic information. Even before the advent of genetic testing, the nation should have held a serious debate about the need for a system to make available a level of coverage to every American who required it. All of us die and there is a long list of ways we might find ourselves with a dependent during our lifetime. Some of these ways are voluntary and optional; some are not. At the time when a person has a dependent, life insurance becomes necessary in most cases.

Because of the complexity of the issue of who really has a dependent, I suggest that all Americans be given the right to secure a guaranteed minimum level of life insurance at standard rates that vary only by age. It would require no health test and no genetic test, and would include a simple questionnaire that would obtain information sufficient to determine only that the person who died was the insured.

The policy would offer a sliding scale of coverage for the first X years (I suggest that $X = 2$ or 3), starting at zero and paying the full policy limit at X years, except in the case of accidental death, for which the full policy benefit would obtain at all times. Coverage would be annual renewal term insurance. The amount I propose is a maximum of $100,000, indexed to inflation at the consumer product index inflation rate from the date of enactment.

The plan would use standard rates plus a small percentage (5% or 10%) that would be based on the average national mortality rate for all persons in the country. A standard commission and overhead and insurer profit margin (based on no risk) would be included. All insurers would offer this coverage at the same rate. Each insurer could offer wrap-around as well as competing plans using fully free-market methods to set the rates and underwrite this business.

Individuals could buy all or some of the first $100,000 on a nonguaranteed basis if they desired. In that case, they would lose the right to buy guaranteed coverage for the level purchased (e.g., if a $50,000 policy was purchased in the free market, the insured would have only a $50,000 right to purchase remaining). This nonguaranteed purchase would be subject to all tests, physical examinations, and questionnaires that the insurer desired to use. A clearing-house on the $100,000 coverage would collect data sufficient to identify if a person ever had the guaranteed coverage or other coverage up to the limit of the guaranteed amount.

Since persons could buy nonguaranteed coverage on a free-market basis, only the standard or better (super-preferred, preferred) risks would do so. This means that guaranteed business at the standard rate would lose money since it would be left with only nonstandard business. All guaranteed business would be pooled in a reinsurance facility. Premiums would be shared as well as losses. The shortfall would be made up by a small surcharge on all life insurance premiums, group and individual.

Individuals would, of course, be free to buy other coverage above the $100,000. The cost would be subject to all requirements the insurer desired to use, including family histories, medical tests, and genetic tests. Purchase of the $100,000 guaranteed coverage would be a one-time right, exercisable at the discretion of the insured. Other proposals would become unnecessary if this primary recommendation were adopted. With a guaranteed layer of coverage, it would not be necessary to prohibit insurance companies from offering preferred rates based on results of genetic tests or genetic information. However, if there were no guaranteed layer, that would be a crucial reform. No doubt "good gene" discounts would drive up prices for the rest of the population, for many to unaffordable levels, and hasten significant segregation of the life insurance market. Similarly, if a guaranteed layer of coverage were in place, with rates set on national averages, it would not be necessary to permit individuals to use results of genetic tests to obtain coverage at regular rates.

Another proposal calls for state legislatures to protect group life insureds (typically groups of employees, whose employer is a sophisticated buyer with considerable market and political clout) but not individual insureds (who typically are not at all sophisticated purchasers and lack both market and political influence). Why should cross-subsidies be acceptable for group life policies but not for individuals?

The proposal made above relies on the idea of a cross-subsidy for a group to which all Americans are potential applicants and all help assure the affordability of guaranteed coverage through a small surcharge on their policies. Permitting genetic information in individual, but not group, policies, besides being adverse to the individual market, would likely reduce availability of small-group policies since small groups would not be broad enough to allay insurer fears of adverse selection.

Several other proposals also should be considered. Particular emphasis should be given to the need to have actuarial, not just genetic, justification for use of genetic information in underwriting. The measure of whether a pricing or underwriting decision is valid is an actuarial not a genetic-scientific one. There must be an actuarial basis for decisions that meet the requirements of the Society of Actuaries and the American Academy of Actuaries.

Another idea is to offer life insurance with no underwriting, but with a five-year waiting period for claims except for accidental death. A form of this concept is adopted in the proposal we put forth above.

Conclusion

Like health insurance, life insurance is a necessity today. Therefore, significant regulatory analysis and control are essential. State legislatures should immediately undertake the important work of reviewing the key question, is life insurance a right in modern America?

A minimum level of life insurance should be assured to all Americans. Procedural and substantive control over the use of genetic information by insurance companies is also required and must be particularly strong if a minimum level of coverage is not guaranteed.

Every person is born with the potential that he or she may be a parent and that illness or death may result in a sudden and unexpected dependent sometime during life. The right to reproduce and to protect loved dependents should not be put at risk in the name of private sector competition. A very small cross-subsidy is a reasonable price to pay to assure the availability of life insurance to all people in America who need it.

References

Consumer Federation of America, Reinventing State Insurance Regulation for the Benefit of Consumers—A Time for Change. Washington, D.C.: Consumer Federation of America (2000).

Consumer Federation of America and National Credit Reporting Association, Credit Score Accuracy and Implications for Consumers. Washington, D.C.: Consumer Federation of America (2002).

Daniels, N., The Functions of Insurance and the Fairness of Genetic Underwriting, in Genetics and Life Insurance: Medical Underwriting and Social Policy, M. A. Rothstein, ed. Cambridge: MIT Press (2004).

Jerry, R. H., Antitrust Implications of Life Insurers' Collaborative Standard Setting, in Genetics and Life Insurance: Medical Underwriting and Social Policy, M. A. Rothstein, ed. Cambridge: MIT Press (2004).

Knoppers, B. M., Godard, B., and Joly, Y., A Comparative, International Overview, in Genetics and Life Insurance: Medical Underwriting and Social Policy, M. A. Rothstein, ed. Cambridge: MIT Press (2004).

MassMutual to Give Away 20,000 Life Insurance Policies to Low-Income Parents, http://info.insure.com/life/mmfreelife902.html (2002).

National Conference of State Legislatures, Genetics and Life, Disability and Long-term Care Insurance. Denver and Washington, D.C.: National Conference of State Legislatures, http://ncsl.org/programs/health/genetics/ndislife.htm (2002).

Rothstein, M. A., Policy Recommendations, in Genetics and Life Insurance: Medical Underwriting and Social Policy, M. A. Rothstein, ed. Cambridge: MIT Press (2004).

11

Policy Recommendations

Mark A. Rothstein

Earlier chapters, individually and collectively, indicated the importance of addressing the issue of the use of genetic information in life insurance underwriting. The life insurance industry plays an enormous economic role in our society. In the United States in 2001, 69% of families maintained some form of life insurance, with a total of over $16 trillion in force (Meyer 2004). Life insurance provides financial security to individuals and families, facilitates attainment of important life goals, such as having children and buying a home, and serves as a vehicle for accumulating assets.

The life insurance industry is built on the principle of risk assessment and classification (Dicke 2004). It is impossible to predict precisely when any currently healthy individual will die. A vigorous, low-risk person may have a heart attack and die tomorrow. A high-risk person, with a dangerous occupation, hobbies, and lifestyle, may live to 100. Life insurance companies, however, do not base their coverage and pricing decisions on individuals, but on groups of individuals. Thus, even if one person's risk of death cannot be determined precisely, actuaries can calculate with a high degree of accuracy the average life expectancy of a group of 1,000 or 10,000 people with similar risks, such as age, current medical conditions (e.g., hypertension, diabetes), and lifestyle factors (e.g., cigarette smoking). Underwriters attempt to place individuals into a category with those of similar risk (Gleeson 2004). Accurate assessment of risk is not only a matter of sound business practice, but so-called "actuarial fairness" in life insurance has been equated with "moral fairness" or justice, in that like cases or risks are treated in an equivalent way (Daniels 2004).

From the perspective of the life insurance industry, the amount of genetic information that increasingly will become available in health care and other settings raises two fundamental questions. First, how can this information be used accurately in medical underwriting, especially when the consequences for life expectancy of newly discovered genetic markers are not clearly understood (Lowden 2004)? Second, how can insurers protect themselves (and policy holders in each risk category) from possible information asymmetry and resulting adverse selection when individual applicants learn of their genetically increased risks for disorders that may not manifest for years, especially when the contestable period is generally two years?

If life insurance companies fear adverse selection, consumers fear genetic discrimination, in which life insurance companies are viewed as invading their privacy and requiring them to confront potentially devastating, predictive genetic information (Hunter 2004). People fear that, on the basis of this information, insurers will either inaccurately assess risks and unjustifiably deny them access to life insurance or charge them excessive rates; or accurately assess risks but unfairly use genetic information to deny them coverage or charge them higher rates for a financial product they need and to which they believe they should have some entitlement (Uhlmann and Terry 2004).

Genetic discrimination in all forms, including life insurance, is widely perceived by the public to be of great concern (Rothstein and Hornung 2004). Moreover, the public believes that insurers' access to and use of genetic information will inevitably lead to negative outcomes for consumers. At the same time, however, many people do not understand the role of genetics in health, the potential benefits of learning predictive genetic information, the risk-classification principles underlying life insurance, or the consequences of adopting various policy options with regard to genetics and life insurance.

One unfortunate health effect of this fear of discrimination (in insurance as well as employment and other areas) is that individuals at risk of genetic disorders, who might be aided by early medical and lifestyle intervention, may decline to undergo genetic testing. Public opinion surveys consistently indicate that at least two-thirds of respondents report that they are less willing to undergo these tests if the results are available to employers, health insurers, or life insurers (Rothstein and Hornung 2004). Thus, the fear of social consequences could lead to adverse population health consequences. Unless this situation is addressed, it would represent a tragic failure of society to take advantage of one of the key benefits of genetic research.

The issue of how, if at all, the law should regulate the use of genetic information in life insurance underwriting has become a point of contention around the world (Knoppers et al. 2004). Proposals to deal with the issue have ranged widely, no doubt influenced by the varying nature and role of life insurance products, the legal environment, tax laws, and cultural attitudes. Various enactments and proposals suggest legislation, a mixture of legislation and insurance industry guidelines, or voluntary measures by the insurance industry. In the United States, however, industry agreements on how to use genetic information in medical underwriting may run afoul of federal and state antitrust laws (Jerry 2004), thus adding one more element of fear.

Current State of the Law

In the United States, as a result of the federal McCarran–Ferguson Act, insurance is generally regulated at the state level, and life insurance is exclusively regulated at the state level (Jerry 2004). Public concerns have led to enactment of laws in nearly all states prohibiting genetic discrimination in health insurance. Although states vary in their definition of "genetic information" and the applicability of the law to individual and small-group policies, they reflect a general consensus that individuals who are asymptomatic should not be excluded from the opportunity to purchase health insurance because of a genetically increased risk of illness. Most people who have health coverage obtain it either through employer-sponsored group plans or federal health programs that are not risk rated (Medicare, Medicaid). Thus, these state laws generally apply only to the 10% of people with individual coverage (National Conference of State Legislatures 2001, p. 12) and the minority of employees with employer-provided, nonself-insured benefits (U.S. Chamber of Commerce 2001, p. 33). Of particular note, these newly enacted state laws neither protect symptomatic individuals (regardless of the cause of their illness) nor prohibit discrimination against applicants based on predictions of future illness attributable to nongenetic factors (Rothstein 1998).

The small amount of empirical evidence available suggests that genetic testing is currently available to only a small segment of the population (Uhlmann and Terry 2004), and that there is little genetic discrimination in health insurance (Hall 1999). It obviously cannot be determined whether discrimination would exist at some time if these laws had not been enacted. Despite lack of a substantial number of documented cases of genetic discrimination in health insurance, it has been relatively easy to forge a political consensus in state legislatures to enact laws offering modest protections to a limited group of individuals without confronting the more contentious, but inextricable, issue of access to health care. As narrowly defined, genetic discrimination in health insurance was an easy target.

The issue of genetic discrimination in life insurance (and disability and long-term care insurance) has not yet been the focus of extensive legislative activity by states, but it may simply be a matter of time before it is; to date, about one-third of states have enacted laws dealing with genetics and life insurance (National Conference of State Legislatures 2002). The laws typically contain one or more of the following provisions: prohibiting unfair genetic discrimination, requiring that genetic information may be used only if it is actuarially justified, and requiring that life insurers obtain informed consent before obtaining results of a genetic test.

These laws provide little new substantive protection for applicants. Unfair trade practice laws in every state already prohibit unfair medical discrimination and require actuarial justification for medical underwriting (Meyer 2004). The problem with these laws is that they generally lack adequate enforcement mechanisms, and insurance commissions and courts tend to give great deference to insurance companies regarding actuarial determinations. In states with informed consent laws, insurers can simply make signing an authorization for release of genetic information a condition of applying for the policy. Thus, state laws have yet to address the fundamental issues of the role of life insurance in our society, the use of genetic information in predicting mortality, and the proper balance of interests of consumers, insurance companies, and the public.

Table 11.1
General Principles for the Use of Genetic Information in Life Insurance

---

1. Do not discourage at-risk individuals from undergoing genetic testing.

2. Do not coerce individuals into undergoing genetic testing.

3. Do not promote harmful social consequences, including genetic reductionism, determinism, and fatalism.

4. Make life insurance coverage available at affordable rates to as many people as possible.

5. Promote actuarially sound underwriting and assure the public that underwriting and pricing decisions are fair.

6. Do not promote or enable adverse selection.

7. Be consistent with current insurance and antitrust laws.

8. Seek to minimize regulatory complexity and costs consistent with achieving key objectives.

9. Anticipate scientific developments.

10. Develop recommendations that are politically feasible.

General Principles

In attempting to devise policies to deal with such a complicated matter, it is valuable to set out general principles to be advanced by the policies. These principles attempt to promote the interests of consumers, insurers, and the public. Because the interests of the parties on some issues are incompatible, it may not be possible to formulate an acceptable strategy that furthers all of the principles. Nevertheless, these general principles provide an analytical starting point. See table 11.1. I previously described some of them in the context of broad public policies dealing with genetics (Rothstein 1997).

1. Do not discourage at-risk individuals from undergoing genetic testing.

The health benefits of genetic research depend on the availability of genetic services and the willingness of individuals to use them. Individuals afflicted with genetic disorders will, no doubt, attempt to obtain therapies to ameliorate the conditions. Those who are asymptomatic, however, are different. Several factors determine whether they decide to have genetic testing, including cost and availability of a medical intervention. For some individuals, the possible social consequences of generating genetic information will discourage them from undergoing presymptomatic testing (Geer et al. 2001). For a few (and presumably increasing number of) disorders, such as colon cancer and breast cancer, timely identification of a genetically increased risk would permit essential medical surveillance or prophylaxis. Public policy should not discourage genetic testing of at-risk individuals (Lowden 2004).

2.   Do not coerce individuals into undergoing genetic testing.

The decision whether to undergo genetic testing, especially for predisposition to serious, adult-onset disorders (those with particular significance for life insurance), is a difficult personal decision with implications for the individual and the individual's family. Genetic counseling long has embraced the model of nondirective, autonomous decision making (Biesecker 1997). In general, public policy should attempt to give effect to this professional standard and therefore should discourage third parties from using economic coercion to compel people to undergo genetic testing.

At the present time, few if any companies require genetic tests as a condition of applying for life insurance. Current tests have too little predictive value and are too expensive to justify their use (Lowden 2004). Nevertheless, it is possible that in a few years multiplex, chip-based tests could be widely available at relatively low cost that would be capable of testing for thousands of mutations simultaneously. Thus, the cost-benefit analysis could change. As discussed below, we must make public policy decisions about whether these tests should be treated differently for regulatory purposes than multiple assay blood tests now widely used by clinicians as well as by insurers.

3.   Do not promote harmful social consequences, including genetic reductionism, determinism, and fatalism.

As individuals learn more about their own genetic makeup, substantial numbers of them are likely to misinterpret the information, potentially leading to serious psychological, social, and societal consequences. Several studies and case reports indicate that many people believe that even complex traits and disorders are attributable to a single gene mutation (genetic reductionism), that having such a mutation invariably leads to gene expression (genetic determinism), and that nothing can be done about it (genetic fatalism) (Wachbroit 2000). People differ widely as to how they express these beliefs, ranging from depression and reclusive risk aversion to mania and reckless risk taking. They also may have feelings of anger, frustration, guilt, or hopelessness. With any extreme reaction, often severe adverse effects occur to the individual, family members (who also may be at risk), and friends and colleagues.

Beyond the need for better education of the public and health professionals about genetics (Andrews et al. 1994, chapter 5) and professional counseling surrounding genetic testing, it is not clear how these concerns translate into effective policies. On the one hand it could be argued that limitations should be placed on generating genetic information that is not essential to a person's health; that less genetic information will minimize the chance of negative social consequences. On the other hand, it could be argued that limitations on generating such information further reinforce the psychological burden of genetic predisposition. Moreover, attempting to limit the amount of genetic information denies individuals positive aspects in terms of medical surveillance and early intervention.

4.   Make life insurance coverage available at affordable rates to as many people as possible.

Although the social significance of life insurance depends on the product (e.g., term insurance, whole life), all forms of life insurance promote important social goals. By providing for income replacement in the event of premature death of the insured, life insurance provides peace of mind to the insured and beneficiaries alike and facilitates their attaining significant life goals such as buying a home and having children.

Despite its clear social value, life insurance is not designed to be a social security system, a welfare system, or a wealth-redistribution system. As presently structured, it is a voluntary, commercial product. It is not available to people who cannot afford the premiums or to those in failing health. The current system would have to be significantly changed (or replaced with a new one) to provide life insurance for the 31% of United States families without coverage.

Thus, the goal of making affordable life insurance available to as many people as possible means that individuals currently offered coverage at standard or preferred rates should continue to be able to obtain that coverage, and as many people as possible who are declined coverage (4.3% of applications) or offered coverage at substandard rates (5% of policies) should be offered coverage at standard or preferred rates. It is not clear to what extent efforts to provide coverage to those currently lacking it will undermine the ability of those who have coverage to maintain it.

5. Promote actuarially sound underwriting and assure the public that underwriting and pricing decisions are fair.

Much of the public concern surrounding the use of genetic information in life insurance underwriting involves the belief that genetic information will be used erroneously by life insurance companies, thereby resulting in unjustified denial of coverage or higher rates. This concern, as it applies to expertise, is not without foundation, as very few physicians, including medical directors of life insurance companies, have formal training in genetics, and the science is changing so quickly that it is difficult to keep abreast of developments. A key challenge, discussed at greater length below, is ensuring the accuracy of medical underwriting. The concern is not well founded, however, if it assumes that genetic information is currently used widely in life insurance underwriting.

6. Do not promote or enable adverse selection.

It is difficult to estimate the degree to which adverse selection would occur if individuals who were at substantially increased genetic risk could obtain life insurance policies at standard rates (Subramanian et al. 1999; Zick et al. 2000). Lack of data, however, does not mean that it would not occur. Home collection genetic test kits are available for several genetic disorders, and increasing availability of testing outside of the clinical setting suggests that at-risk individuals can learn their genotype in off-record testing.

Information asymmetry satisfies the first half of the formula for adverse selection. The second half is the inclination of consumers to act on the basis of the greater information. As discussed in chapter 1, our nationwide consumer survey indicated that 23.1% strongly agreed and 50% agreed that consumers would withhold unfavorable results of a genetic test from a life insurance company. Other evidence confirms this view. Nonsmokers have better rates on life insurance than smokers; however, to verify their nonsmoking status, insurers test urine or oral fluid samples for the presence of cotinine, the metabolite of nicotine. According to data from LABOne, the largest laboratory performing these tests, 7% to 14% of declared nonsmokers tested positive for coti-nine, thereby indicating that they had mischaracterized themselves.

If adverse selection based on genetic test results were to occur, the effects could be significant in terms of cost shifting to low-risk policy holders and the financial viability of insurers. Some level of adverse selec-tion undoubtedly already exists in many insurance product lines, and it is probably priced into the product. Nevertheless, it is important to con-sider whether policy recommendations regarding genetic information would increase the likelihood of adverse selection in life insurance.

7. Be consistent with current insurance and antitrust laws.

Because life insurance is regulated by states, it will likely be necessary to develop model language or consensus policies to effect a change in every jurisdiction. In addition, federal and state antitrust laws may be implicated by life insurance practices. For example, a voluntary agree-ment by life insurance companies dealing with genetic information could be considered a restraint of trade and therefore unlawful under antitrust law. Policy recommendations should take into account this legislative framework.

8. Seek to minimize regulatory complexity and costs consistent with achieving key objectives.

The simplicity, efficiency, and ease of administration of a proposal should be considered in any policy enactment. All things being equal, the simplest alternative will better serve the interests of consumers, insurers, regulators, and the public.

9. Anticipate scientific developments.

The science of genetics is changing virtually daily, and public policy should anticipate scientific advances. For example, it is not enough to say that few if any life insurance companies are performing genetic tests today. Nor is it enough to say that we have little evidence that adverse selection is taking place by individuals who have genetic informa-tion that is not known by insurers. Trends are toward developing more diagnostic and predictive tests, lowering the cost of testing, increasing the predictive value of testing, and expanding consumer access to test-ing (possibly including a large increase in home-collection test kits).

Therefore, policies must anticipate an increase in the volume of testing as well as other factors.

10.   Develop recommendations that are politically feasible.

As if the first nine principles were not daunting enough, recommendations should, at least, have a chance of being enacted. For example, chances are extremely remote that political support exists for a generous, government-sponsored benefit program for survivors or government-subsidized, high-limit life insurance without medical underwriting. Similarly, it must be assumed that policies requiring a major restructuring of commercial life insurance are not politically feasible.

Genetic Exceptionalism

An extremely important, but as yet unresolved, issue of public policy is whether genetic information should be treated the same as other medical information. It has come to be known as the debate over "genetic exceptionalism." One of the first expert groups to study the issue of genetic information and insurance was the Task Force on Genetic Information and Insurance of the NIH-DOE Joint Working Group on the Ethical, Legal, and Social Implications of the Human Genome Project. "The task force used the term genetic exceptionalism to mean roughly the claim that genetic information is sufficiently different from other kinds of health-related information that it deserves special protection or other exceptional measures" (Murray 1997). Ultimately, for both moral and practical reasons, the task force rejected the notion of treating genetic information differently.

It is important to review the reasons cited by both proponents and opponents of genetic-specific laws. Those in favor of genetic-specific laws generally rely on the following arguments:

1. Genetic information is unique because it may reveal information about family members as well as the individual.
2. Genetic information is unique because it may have implications for reproduction and characteristics of future generations.
3. Genetic information is unique because it may be predictive.
4. Genetic information often carries stigma, and in the past its misuse led to eugenics, racism, and genocide.

5. Genetic information is regarded as unique by the public.

6. Other special categories of medical information exist for which separate protections have been adopted, including HIV infection and mental illness.

7. The political reality is that genetic nondiscrimination laws have greater support than more general, and seemingly more sweeping, legislation.

Opponents of genetic-specific laws generally rely on the following arguments:

1. It is difficult to make a moral argument that it is impermissible to discriminate against people on the basis of genetic information, but that it is permissible to discriminate against them on the basis of other medical information.

2. Intractable problems are associated with defining "genetic" because the definitions are either too narrow (including only results of a DNA-based test, many people can be subject to discrimination based on family health histories) or too broad (including family histories and complex disorders, virtually all medical conditions would be covered).

3. It is impossible to separate genetic information from other medical information in medical records.

4. A general law is easier for individuals and affected entities to comply with.

5. By having the same laws applicable to all forms of medical information, the stigma of genetic information would be diminished rather than reinforced.

From a scientific standpoint, if there ever was a time when genetic and nongenetic diseases could be neatly divided, that time is long past. It is clear that both genetic and environmental factors are involved in virtually every malady. For example, many monogenic disorders require a particular environmental condition before they will be expressed. Conversely, even with prototypically environmental illnesses, such as infectious diseases, genetic factors play a role in susceptibility or resistance, the course of the illness, and the most efficacious pharmaceutical therapies. Thus, it makes little sense to persist with a political dichotomy at a time when science no longer recognizes or supports such a clear distinction.

Genetic exceptionalism is criticized by most commentators (Lemmens 2000; Murray 1997; Rothstein 1999), but it has received the support of state legislatures, primarily through enactment of laws prohibiting genetic discrimination in employment and health insurance as well as more general genetic-privacy laws. Unless thinking undergoes a substantial change, it is reasonable to assume that, to the extent that the use of genetic information in life insurance is regulated, it will take place through enactment of genetic-specific laws. Yet, only political expediency militates in favor of such an approach. Current genetic-specific laws for health insurance and employment have not been effective for both theoretical and practical reasons (Rothstein 1998), and similar enactments with regard to life insurance are also likely to fail. This is a point of agreement between many advocates of life insurance underwriting reform and the life insurance industry, which opposes genetic-specific laws. The difficult issue, of course, is to shape the contours of new regulation that would further the public policy goals set out above that are fair and capable of garnering the support of all sides.

Procedural Reforms

The use of predictive medical information (including predictive genetic information) for nonmedical purposes (including medical underwriting in life insurance) gives rise to three concerns of individuals: (1) the predictions may be inaccurate; (2) the information generated in making the predictions also may be used for other purposes; or (3) the predictions will be accurate, but may lead to adverse economic or social consequences.

Some in the industry contend that because life insurance is so competitive, an individual who is declined or offered a policy at substandard rates by one insurer should merely apply to another company. This is considered preferable to new regulations and appeal processes. Procedural reforms are unnecessary, the argument goes, because market forces will work to the advantage of consumers, much the way it does when one shops for the best price and terms on a new car or other product.

The analogy to buying consumer products is inapt, however, because, compared with other sales and services, the insurance industry is more heavily regulated, life insurance has greater social significance, and the process of underwriting and pricing life insurance involves personal (including medical) information and increasingly technical-scientific mat-

Table 11.2
Procedural Reforms

1. Regulate use of predictive medical tests
2. Regulate testing laboratories
3. Regulate medical decision makers
4. Require informed consent for all medical examinations and tests
5. Require life insurers to disclose the medical basis of an adverse underwriting decision
6. Provide a right to appeal an adverse underwriting decision
7. Prohibit use of medical information across insurance product lines or to underwrite family members

ters. Therefore, it is appropriate for policy makers to enact additional measures to regulate procedures surrounding the use of medical information in life insurance underwriting to establish greater transparency, regularity, and accountability. Not only must underwriting and pricing be fair in fact, but the public must be assured that they are fair. Thus at-risk individuals will not decline valuable predictive testing or engage in defensive practices to avoid what many consumers might consider to be the erroneous or unfair use of medical information. Although many life insurance companies already follow some or all of the procedures recommended below (summarized in table 11.2), public anxiety suggests the need to regularize the process.

1. Regulate use of predictive medical tests.

Inaccurate predictions based on results of a medical test can be caused by limitations of the test, laboratory errors, or interpretive errors. Lack of regulation in all three areas has been questioned in clinical application of genetic tests, and these problems will have to be resolved regarding genetic information for medical underwriting in life insurance. With regard to the predictive value of genetic tests, both the Institute of Medicine (Andrews et al. 1994) and the Task Force on Genetic Testing (Holtzman and Watson 1998) observed that there is little regulation of the genetic testing industry. In some instances, tests are developed and marketed (often directly to consumers) before adequate evidence of analytical validity, clinical validity, or clinical utility is available. Most tests are performed to determine the presence of an allele associated with a greater risk of illness. Such tests, even if accurate in the sense that they correctly identify the mutation (analytical validity), still have little value unless a correlation is found between the mutation and a discernible risk of developing a phenotypic response, taking into account the degree of penetrance and the variability of expression (clinical validity).

To be valuable for medical underwriting in life insurance, a test result must be linked with a statistically significant increased risk of developing a potentially lethal, adult-onset disorder, and clinical or actuarial data of the effect of the mutation on mortality risk must exist. As most genetic tests were developed in the past decade, little mortality data are available except for those derived by extrapolation. With the shift in research focus from monogenic to complex disorders, environmental influences will become increasingly important but difficult to factor into mortality calculations. Furthermore, the longer the latency period before onset of symptoms, the more speculative the estimate of mortality risk becomes, because of inability to predict intervening medical discoveries that could ameliorate the condition and thereby change mortality calculations. All of these factors make it clear that even tests with clinical utility, because they are valuable in lifestyle modifications or medical surveillance, may have only limited value in medical underwriting for life insurance (Lowden 2004).

In theory, medical underwriters would not require tests that were not proved to be predictive because such tests would not be worth the cost to insurers. The cost factor, however, does not pertain to tests that were performed in the clinical setting and disclosed pursuant to an authorization. The increasing availability of genetic test results at no cost to insurers raises the possibility of erroneous reliance on questionable tests by at least some companies. Thus, it is important to safeguard the public interest in restricting the use of unproved tests as well as to reassure the public that inappropriate tests will not be used in medical underwriting. As long as life insurance companies are not overly restricted in using traditional tests, it is hard to imagine their opposition to a ban on newly developed tests lacking scientific evidence. From the industry point of view, the problem would be how to dispense with dubious tests without adding needless costs and bureaucracy and not undermining established practices.

State legislatures should authorize their insurance commissions to publish annual lists of diagnostic and predictive tests that were approved or not approved for medical underwriting. To aid in making such determinations, the National Association of Insurance Commissioners should appoint a medical underwriting advisory committee comprised of medical experts, consumer representatives, and insurance representatives. The committee would be charged with adding tests to and removing them from a national listing. The list would not include cut-off levels or permissible uses of the information in underwriting. These actions would then be reviewed by regulators at the state level.

A committee with a comparable mission was established by the Association of British Insurers (ABI). In the United States, having underwriting standards codified by state governments avoids possible antitrust problems, and having broad representation on the committee assures the public that diverse interests are represented. Furthermore, the list of approved tests would be a public document available to all consumers.

2.   Regulate testing laboratories.

A medical test is only as good as the laboratory performing it. Much has been written about the fact that laboratories performing genetic tests are minimally regulated, especially in light of the high complexity of many tests. Although all laboratories providing information for the diagnosis, prevention, or treatment of human disease are required to comply with the Clinical Laboratories Improvement Amendments of 1988 (CLIA88), no specific requirements apply to genetic tests (Holtzman and Watson 1997, chapter 3). Because these tests have no mandatory proficiency standards, "[f]ew laboratories performing genetic tests as their sole or principal activity are yet complying with the CLIA88 regulations" (Andrews et al. 1994, p. 126). Moreover, regulations issued under CLIA88 are aimed at assuring analytical validity and quality assurance. They do not address clinical validity or clinical utility (Secretary's Advisory Committee on Genetic Testing 2000). In addition, "in-house" or "home brew" (individually developed) tests often differ among laboratories and are not subject to regulation.

State legislation should be enacted to require that all medical tests performed in the process of medical underwriting for life insurance be performed in a laboratory certified under CLIA, a laboratory certified by a state agency in a CLIA-exempt jurisdiction such as New York or Washington, or a laboratory certified by the College of American Pathologists or other professional organization performing regular proficiency testing. Although most insurance testing already is performed in a certified laboratory, a statutory requirement of certification will assure the public that tests are performed properly.

3.   Regulate medical decision makers.

Vast numbers of physicians lack the education or training to understand the field of medical genetics. Numerous studies confirm the inadequacy of medical school curricula in genetics, especially for physicians who graduated from medical school before 1970 (Holtzman and Watson 1997, chapter 4). In one study, over one-third of family physicians who did not deliver babies, internists, and psychiatrists had scores of 65% correct or lower on a series of genetics questions deemed important by a panel of nongeneticist providers (Hofman et al. 1993). The only study on knowledge of genetics by insurance physicians was published in 1993, and it concluded that the physicians may lack the knowledge necessary to make increasingly complex predictions of mortality risk based on genetic information (McEwen et al. 1993). According to a study in the United Kingdom (Low et al. 1998), some life insurers using genetic information erroneously excluded applicants from coverage, including unaffected carriers of recessive disorders and parents of children who had a genetic disorder caused by a spontaneous mutation. Even though it is still the case that few insurance physicians have formal training in genetics, the topic is now more frequently discussed at professional meetings and in the insurance medicine literature than it was in the early 1990s.

Although there is no legal requirement that life insurance companies must employ physicians to provide advice on medical underwriting policy, all large insurers and reinsurers have physicians working for them. In midsize companies this may be a part-time consultant. Small companies either have a part-time consultant or rely on reinsurers for medical underwriting. Physicians who have been in insurance medicine for four years are eligible to take written and oral examinations in insurance medicine offered by the Board of Insurance Medicine. Those who pass the examinations are board certified. Past written examinations had only a limited number of questions on genetics, but the 2003 version had greater emphasis on the subject. The American Academy of Insurance Medicine is approved as a member of the American Medical Association's House of Delegates. As of October 2002, 321 board-certified insurance physicians were in active practice, including Canadian and European members. With some large insurance companies having more than one board-certified physician, and more than 1,500 life insurance companies in North America, most companies lack a board-certified physician on a full-time or part-time basis.

To ensure that medical underwriting decisions are made by properly trained individuals, state laws or insurance regulations should be enacted to require, at a minimum, that all such decisions be made by or under the supervision of a licensed physician. Further regulation, such as requiring board certification, would have to be phased in, given the low numbers of certified individuals. Expert consultants also should be required for underwriting cases involving specialized or complex areas of medicine.

4.   Require informed consent for all medical examinations and tests.

Physicians who examine and perform medical tests on patients are required to obtain informed consent. Among other things, patients must be informed of the purpose of all procedures, risks and benefits, alternatives, and findings. The legal basis for informed consent is the physician-patient relationship. However, when a physician examines an individual on behalf of and for the benefit of a third party (including an insurance company) merely to assess the individual's health status and no treatment is contemplated, no physician-patient relationship exists (Rothstein 1984). Therefore, common law duties associated with a physician-patient relationship do not apply. The physician is required only to obtain consent to touch the person in the course of the examination, and generally incurs liability only for physically injuring the person during the examination.

Medical examinations and tests performed in the course of applying for life insurance have significant, potential social and psychological consequences. Despite absence of a common law physician-patient relationship, every person should have a statutory right to be told for whom the physician works, the nature of tests to be performed, findings indicating an adverse health risk, and other matters in the process of providing informed consent.

5.   Require life insurers to disclose the medical basis of an adverse underwriting decision.

Unknown numbers of life insurance companies have a policy of notifying individuals of the medical reason for denial of coverage or the offer of a policy at substandard rates; yet, few if any states have made this a legal requirement. Typically, the only applicable legislation requires an insurer or testing laboratory to report to the state health department the names of individuals who test positive for hepatitis B, hepatitis C, or HIV. The purpose of such disclosure is to promote public health and not to advance consumer protection.

To promote accountability in life insurance underwriting, state legislatures should enact laws requiring life insurers to notify applicants of the basis for a decision denying coverage or offering a policy at substandard rates. A few states, such as New York and Maine, have notification requirements applicable only to results of genetic tests. Because substandard offers may be based on occupation, recreation activities, or international travel, in addition to medical reasons, notification of the reason for an adverse decision is essential.

6.   Provide a right to appeal an adverse underwriting decision.

On receiving notice of the reason for denial of coverage or an offer at substandard rates, a person should have a right to appeal the decision. This appeal could be within the insurance company, if an adequate procedure is established. In any event, adverse decisions should be appealable to the state insurance commissioner or some other individual or body established to review the sufficiency of medical evidence on which the adverse action is based. State laws also should mandate that consumers be informed about their right to appeal adverse decisions and the procedure for doing so, because few consumers are aware of their rights when they exist (Uhlmann and Terry 2004).

Few insurance commissions or departments have the jurisdiction or inclination to review individual underwriting decisions. Permitting such review would be analogous to independent review of health insurance coverage and claims decisions, now the law in virtually every state (Mariner 2002). Despite considerable opposition from insurers and health maintenance organizations when these laws were originally enacted, appeals have been invoked infrequently (American Political

Network 2002) and the laws are generally praised by consumers and at least tolerated by the industry. After exhausting the administrative process, aggrieved persons should have the right to bring a private action in court to review the decision of the independent review board. Then if successful, the person should be entitled to purchase the policy from the insurer to which the application was made at a rate commensurate with the risk, and to receive the costs of the appeal, including reasonable attorney fees. Statutory damages should be recoverable only on a showing that the decision was arbitrary and capricious. The insurance commission also should have the ability to sanction insurance companies shown to exhibit a pattern of unlawful conduct in underwriting.

Some states with unfair trade practice laws prohibiting unfair discrimination provide for a private right of action, but most states do not recognize an individual's ability to bring such claims (Ostrager and Newman 2000). Similarly, the courts have rejected arguments that the actuarially unsupported denial of a life insurance policy constitutes actionable disability discrimination under the public accommodations title of the Americans with Disabilities Act (*Chabner v. United of Omaha Life Insurance Co.* 2000). Thus, without enacting specific new legislation, people will continue to have little legal redress to challenge medical underwriting decisions.

As a practical matter, relatively few individuals are likely to appeal. With numerous life insurers aggressively competing for business, after a denial or offer of coverage at substandard rates, it may be easier for the applicant to seek insurance from another insurer. Nevertheless, it is important to have a procedure in place to encourage fairness in decision making.

7.   Prohibit use of medical information across insurance product lines and to underwrite family members.

Another concern is that genetic information obtained by an insurer for one purpose will be used for another purpose. With companies frequently offering more than one insurance line, it would be possible for them to rely on information obtained in an application for life insurance to be applied to disability or long-term care insurance. Similarly, because of the familial nature of genetic risk, many are concerned that genetic information obtained in the medical underwriting of one family member will be used in the consideration of other family members.

To address both of these concerns, state legislatures should enact laws prohibiting insurance companies from using medical information across product lines and to underwrite family members. Some states already have laws prohibiting the use of genetic test results of family members in underwriting (e.g., New York, Vermont). Similarly, the Code of Practice of the Association of British Insurers provides that "genetic information relating to one family member will not be linked or transferred to applications for insurance made by another family member" (Cook 1999). The Investment and Financial Services Association of Australia also adopted such a rule (2002). In Kansas, insurers are prohibited from using genetic information across product lines. Even a more general law, applicable to all medical information, would not prohibit life insurance companies from asking customary questions about family health history. Consequently, the practical effect of such enactments may be limited, but the laws may prevent some at-risk individuals from declining to undergo genetic testing.

Substantive Options

The preceding part of this chapter discussed several possible procedural reforms for underwriting in life insurance. Specifically, it addressed ways of ensuring the accuracy of predictive mortality calculations as well as ways of limiting the use of medical information. The remaining policy issue is certainly the most difficult, and it is the substantive question of whether the current underwriting system and pricing structure of life insurance should be changed in any way. The role of genetic and other factors in life expectancy is a factual matter. The way we permit individuals to be aggregated for underwriting purposes, however, is a value and policy judgment of society.

In addressing these issues, it may be valuable to consider the case of health (or medical expense) insurance. Norman Daniels (2004) made the argument that because access to a reasonable level of health care depends on access to private health insurance, compelling moral reasons exist for prohibiting the operation of a purely market-based system of private health insurance. In other words, even though risk-based health insurance may be actuarially fair (in the sense that the risk assessment is accurate), it is not morally fair because it denies access to a fundamentally important social good.

In determining whether a similar analysis should be applied to life insurance it is necessary to consider the moral mission of life insurance. If it is considered a purely commercial transaction, even though it may be regulated by the state, the fundamental underwriting and pricing function should not be altered as long as it is actuarially fair and health information is not used for other purposes. (Procedural recommendations earlier in this chapter addressed these issues.)

On the other hand, if providing or subsidizing a death benefit to survivors is deemed an essential public policy, the goal can be accomplished in two ways. First, it can be considered an entitlement and directly administered by the government. Under Social Security, surviving spouses and dependent children are entitled to benefits based on the decedent's lifetime earnings. For example, if a forty-year-old earning $50,000 per year died today, the surviving spouse would receive $16,596 per year and a surviving child would receive $12,624, with an annual family maximum of $29,248. In addition, they receive a one-time burial benefit of $255 (Social Security Administration 2002). Greater benefits could be funded by increased Social Security contributions or other taxes. Although protection would be expanded by providing coverage to individuals who cannot currently afford life insurance, the costs could be enormous, and the benefits would remain employment based. Second, while retaining the existing private life insurance structure, legislation could be enacted so that individuals who are denied life insurance or charged higher rates because of medical risks would be able to obtain coverage at affordable rates.

It is unlikely that legislators will enact new taxes to fund a more generous government death benefit for survivors. It is also possible that state legislatures will restrict their activity to those procedural issues discussed previously. Nevertheless, judging from activity in Europe (Knoppers et al. 2004) and increasing numbers of bills introduced in state legislatures each year on the issue, many states will eventually take substantive action.

Earlier in this chapter, I made a case against genetic exceptionalism. Nevertheless, many proposals in the literature and in unenacted bills introduced in state legislatures to address the use of genetic information

Table 11.3
Leading Substantive Options

---

1. Establish a moratorium on requiring genetic testing and use of genetic information

2. Prohibit genetic testing and using genetic information

3. Prohibit insurers from requiring genetic testing, but permit use of genetic information

4. Establish a maximum amount of coverage that can be obtained without genetic testing or genetic information

5. Prohibit insurance companies from offering preferred rates based on results of genetic tests or genetic information

6. Permit individuals to use results of genetic tests to obtain coverage at regular rates

7. Prohibit use of predictive testing or predictive information in group life insurance

8. Establish high-risk life insurance pools

9. Other proposals

---

in medical underwriting for life insurance are genetic specific. To make the analysis of the options consistent with the actual proposals, I will consider the proposals as genetic specific where appropriate. Other options (summarized in table 11.3) are presented as more generally applicable to predictive testing and predictive information.

1. Establish a moratorium on requiring genetic testing and use of genetic information.

A moratorium could be imposed legislatively or voluntarily by individual insurers. There is no agreement on the length of time for the moratorium, although five years is frequently mentioned. Moratoria already have been adopted in some countries, including France, Germany, and the United Kingdom (Knoppers et al. 2004).

The theory behind a moratorium is that scientific and policy issues will be clarified in the next few years and appropriate policies can then be determined. From a scientific standpoint, this is wishful thinking. Although the relationship between some genotypes and mortality risks may be better established, the basic scientific issue—use of genetic information when its actuarial significance is not definitively established—will remain. As scientists accumulate better data on some associations, other associations will be suspected and investigated. Thus, the uncertainty simply will be shifted to a different group of genetic variations. With regard to policy, the question of the degree to which life insurance underwriting and pricing should be regulated to promote social considerations will remain the same.

It might seem that a moratorium is valuable in preserving the status quo of little or no genetic testing or use of genetic information in life insurance until better scientific information is available and more detailed policy debates can take place. A moratorium, however, is not a neutral way to buy time. By endorsing the feasibility and acceptability of underwriting without considering genetic information, a moratorium declares the desirability of genetic-free underwriting. Furthermore, once a moratorium is in effect it may be difficult to remove. Consequently, it must be considered the equivalent of legislation banning genetic testing and/or use of genetic information.

2.   Prohibit genetic testing and using genetic information.

At first glance, prohibiting insurers from requiring genetic testing and using genetic information would appear to be the most effective way to "avoid the creation of an uninsurable underclass of individuals" (National Conference of State Legislatures 2001, p. 36). By prohibiting use of genetic information, however, family health histories and other traditional measures of risk assessment also would be prohibited. As a result, major changes would be required in the way life insurance is underwritten and priced.

This option highlights the problem of genetic-specific approaches. A narrow definition of "genetic" to include only results of a DNA-based test is underinclusive and offers no protection against adverse treatment based on family health risks. Furthermore, it affords greater protection to individuals who have a genetic risk than to those with other medical risks. A broader definition of "genetic" to include family health information would, in effect, ban all underwriting and change life insurance to a guaranteed-issue product.

3.   Prohibit insurers from requiring genetic testing, but permit use of genetic information.

Under this option individuals would not be compelled to undergo insurer-ordered genetic testing as a condition of applying for life insurance. Insurers, however, could use the results of genetic tests already performed and in a person's medical record. This compromise option raises problems for both insurance companies and consumers. For insurers, individuals who were tested in research studies, anonymously, or off the record would be able to apply for life insurance without any way for underwriters to know of the results of the test. This is a recipe for adverse selection. Individuals, however, would not do well under this approach either. They would be deterred from having genetic testing in the health care setting, where it would be most beneficial, because the results would be placed in their medical record. Moreover, even without such test results, persons at increased risk because of family health history would still be subject to higher rates or denial of coverage.

Advocates of prohibiting life insurers from requiring genetic testing also must deal with another fundamental issue. If companies are permitted to require some medical tests (e.g., cholesterol, HIV, hepatitis B and C), on what basis should genetic tests be treated differently? (Concern that the tests are insufficiently predictive will be addressed by procedural reforms mentioned earlier.) Assuming the tests are predictive, does something inherent in the fact that they are genetic suggest they should not be used?

Although undoubtedly some stigma are attached to genetic information, this is likely to change within a decade. Genetic information is likely to lose its special or unusual quality, as increased amounts of it will be developed in routine medical care and will be in virtually everyone's medical file. Another important consideration is that irrespective of current stigma, genetic information is not confined to a racial, ethnic, or gender group. Therefore, genetic testing is not analogous to race-based underwriting, which has been prohibited for decades on policy grounds. Indeed, gender is still a lawful and socially acceptable basis for different pricing in life insurance. It is hard to argue that predictive genetic tests (assuming they could be defined) should be prohibited, but that other forms of predictive medical tests should remain permissible. Public anxiety surrounding genetics should be addressed through education and more general privacy and consumer-protection laws, and should not be reinforced by well-meaning but flawed genetic-specific laws.

4.   Establish a maximum amount of coverage that can be obtained without genetic testing or genetic information.

Establishment of maximum levels of coverage without genetic test results or other genetic information (sometimes referred to as a "safe harbor" or a "monetary threshold" approach) is popular in Western Europe, and some attempts have been made to introduce similar legislation in the United States. In Europe, however, life insurance has a different social role, because it is essential to have life insurance to obtain a mortgage. It is a different product with a different public interest at stake.

In European countries that adopted this approach, about $100,000 is the lowest level of life insurance coverage available without genetic testing or consideration of genetic information. With the average policy in the United States in 2000 of $134,800 (Meyer 2004), a substantial percentage of the market would be included under a comparable proviso. In practice, establishing maximum levels of coverage without genetic information would be difficult. First, it would be necessary to define "genetic." Does the prohibition apply only to genetic testing or does it also apply to genetic information? As discussed previously, either definition raises serious problems. Second, it would be necessary to have some way of determining whether people had policies from more than one insurance company so that those at risk could not obtain a series of policies below the maximum (Rothstein 1993). Third, some market adjustments in pricing would be necessary. For example, if companies could not consider genetic information in underwriting policies of $100,000 or less, the rates for a $110,000 policy for a low-risk person (using genetic information) would likely be lower than for a $100,000 policy in the all-applicant (not using genetic information) pool. This would encourage individuals to undergo genetic testing, and then apply for the higher amount if they tested negative and the lower amount if they tested positive. This would increase the price disparity between the genetically underwritten and nonunderwritten pools in a spiraling fashion. Thus, additional regulation or subsidies would be necessary to adjust the pricing structure.

5.   Prohibit insurance companies from offering preferred rates based on results of genetic tests or genetic information.

One scenario in which life insurance companies may be compelled by market forces to require genetic testing or use genetic information is the following. Company A begins to offer a "good gene" discount of 25%

on its life insurance to individuals who voluntarily take ten selected genetic tests and are found not to have any deleterious mutations. Low-risk individuals will flock to company A for the discount. Company B, having lost some of its low-risk insureds, will then be forced either to raise rates for remaining policy holders and new applicants or also use genetic tests. This could quickly put pressure on other companies to do the same and, eventually, the rest of the industry would become segmented by whether genetic information was used.

Although it is not clear that the science would currently justify such an adjustment in the pricing structure merely based on the absence of ten deleterious mutations (Lowden 2004), the possibility of at least some companies attempting this approach cannot be dismissed. To prevent this from occurring, legislation could be enacted to prohibit life insurance companies from using the results of genetic tests or genetic information to sell policies at preferred rates (below standard). This is now expressly permitted under Indiana law, whereas Oregon prohibits the use of favorable genetic information to induce the sale of insurance. The Code of Practice of the Association of British Insurers, however, provides that "insurers will not offer cheaper than normal (standard) premiums to individuals who are perceived to have a good genetic profile" (Cook 1999). A similar policy was adopted by IFSA (2002). Individuals who qualify for preferred rates independent of genetic information would not be affected by this proposal.

6. Permit individuals to use results of genetic tests to obtain coverage at regular rates.

An insurance company that is not permitted to use results of genetic tests would be forced to charge higher premiums to an individual who had a familial risk of a serious illness, but who had undergone genetic testing and learned that he or she did not inherit the lethal mutation. To prevent this from occurring, it has been suggested (and actually enacted in some states) that people should be allowed to use the results of genetic tests if they are favorable.

To prevent the assessment spiral from occurring, as well as coercing individuals into genetic testing, the individual should be permitted to obtain coverage at the regular rate he or she would be offered if genetic information were not considered. Thus, genetic information could not be the basis for a preferred rate, but a preferred rate could be offered to someone with a negative genetic test who would otherwise qualify for a preferred rate for other reasons, such as nonsmoking and healthy lifestyle.

This option operates as an exception to legislation prohibiting use of genetic information in underwriting. If insurers were permitted to use genetic information they could use both favorable and unfavorable data and the exception would be unnecessary.

7.   Prohibit use of predictive testing or predictive information in group life insurance.

About one-third of all life insurance policies are purchased by employers or associations or as credit insurance under group policies (National Conference of State Legislatures 2001, p. 26). In theory, the group is underwritten, but individuals in the group are not. Nevertheless, there is some degree of medical underwriting in group life insurance, depending on the size and nature of the group.

Legislatures should prohibit use of predictive medical information in group life insurance. A similar measure was enacted to deal with medical underwriting in group health insurance as part of the federal Health Insurance Portability and Accountability Act of 1996. Such a measure might increase the price of group life insurance slightly, but only to the extent that underwriting takes place in group policies.

It is important to justify prohibiting medical underwriting in group policies while permitting it in individual policies. The key is the risk of adverse selection. Group life insurance carries less risk of adverse selection because group policies tend to have lower coverage amounts, and the groups (employee groups) are formed for reasons other than to obtain life insurance. The proposed prohibition would not apply to "buy-up" arrangements in group policies, where individuals elect to increase their coverage from the base level, as well as late entrants and reentrants. This approach is used in group disability insurance, where buy-up policies are individually underwritten because of the tendency of less healthy individuals to seek additional coverage.

8.   Establish high-risk life insurance pools.

Previous options attempted to make adjustments to the current system of medical underwriting to prevent insurers from considering an individual's genetically increased risk of illness. If the ultimate goal of legislation dealing with genetic (or predictive) information is to provide an opportunity for high-risk individuals to purchase life insurance at affordable rates, it is better to confront the issue directly. The most likely way of ensuring access to life insurance is to create high-risk pools. These are already established in various other insurance product lines, including health, auto, and workers' compensation insurance. The efficacy of a reinsurance pool was explored by the United Kingdom Human Genetics Commission (2001). In the United States, if public policy supports taxpayer subsidization of flood insurance for beachfront vacation homes, some subsidies should be possible for life insurance for high-risk individuals.

High-risk pools could operate in various ways, but basically the rates of high-risk individuals would be subsidized by low-risk individuals, taxpayers (through a government-supported reinsurance pool), or some combination of subsidies. Many details would have to be worked out, including subsidy amounts, coverage amounts, health status eligibility criteria, timing for purchase, and cost. If we are committed to making life insurance more widely available, however, consumer groups, insurance industry leaders, and public officials must give high-risk pools careful consideration. The first step could be to establish a joint task force consisting of state legislative officials, state insurance commissioners, actuaries, economists, life insurance medical directors, life insurance industry executives, and consumer representatives. This task force could explore the range of options for high-risk pools and develop concrete proposals.

9.   Other proposals.

Several other proposals have been suggested in the literature and draft legislation, including the following: (1) maintain the status quo; (2) require informed consent for insurer-mandated genetic testing; (3) require actuarial justification for use of genetic information in underwriting; (4) prohibit denials, but permit price adjustments based on genetic information; (5) adjust premiums based on willingness to share genetic information, with less information meaning higher premiums; (6) offer condition-specific products at an increased premium to reflect higher risk; and (7) offer life insurance policies with no medical underwriting, but with a five-year waiting period except in the case of accidental death.

The feasibility and desirability of these proposals were addressed directly or indirectly in discussing the other options. These other proposals are less likely to be enacted and less desirable than previous ones. Two of the most seemingly attractive options are the ones to require actuarial justification and to offer life insurance policies with no medical underwriting but with a five-year exclusion period. As to the first, similar unfair trade practice laws are already in effect in every state, but without additional substantive or procedural enactments, a specific provision for genetics adds little or no protection. For the second, policies with no medical underwriting and five-year exclusion periods would not work unless all life insurance were offered in this manner, because adverse selection and pricing would segment the market into immediate and delayed coverage.

Conclusion

The legislative focus on genetic discrimination in insurance is shifting from health insurance to life insurance. Policy development for life insurance will be more difficult than for health insurance. Life insurance is regarded by the public as less essential than health insurance (Rothstein and Hornung 2004), and therefore less sweeping regulatory intervention is likely. It still plays an important societal role, however, and labeling it as a commercial transaction does not mean that market efficiency should take precedence over the more abstract interests of autonomy, beneficence, privacy, and well-being.

After enacting numerous laws to regulate use of genetic information in health insurance, state legislatures are turning their attention to life insurance. In the absence of a comprehensive and coherent approach to medical underwriting in life insurance, the states have begun (and are likely to continue) to enact a patchwork of genetic-specific laws. These laws attempt to address procedural, substantive, and privacy issues while treating genetic information separately from other medical information. The limits of these approaches suggest the need for policy makers to consider a range of new approaches.

In reviewing substantive options, it should be clear that there is no free lunch. If life insurance for high-risk individuals is to be made available at below actuarially determined rates, a subsidy must come from another source, either low-risk individuals or taxpayers. Perhaps the greatest challenge is to enact policies with the fewest unintended consequences. One way to minimize such consequences is to attack the problem directly. Temporizing strategies, such as moratoria and prohibiting insurers from requiring genetic testing but permitting them to use results of prior genetic tests and family health histories, are likely to make matters worse. Indeed, no genetic-specific law is likely to be effective. Genetic tests and information are nearly impossible to define or isolate in medical records; enacting genetic-specific laws also reinforces stigma.

The three main parties of interest are faced with important challenges. First, the life insurance industry must recognize the depth of concern among the public indicated in the survey data in chapter 1. It should support procedural reforms, such as those detailed here, to bring greater transparency and accountability to underwriting and pricing, thereby assuring the public that medical underwriting is fair and that medical information will not be used for other purposes. The industry also should be willing to support substantive measures, such as prohibiting offering policies at preferred rates based on genetic information, banning underwriting in group policies, and establishing high-risk life insurance pools.

Second, the public must not expect something for nothing. It must develop a better understanding of genetics as well as the principles of life insurance. If the consensus is that life insurance should be made available to high-risk individuals, a realistic discussion of the costs involved and allocation of those costs must take place.

Finally, legislators must be willing to consider the more difficult and complicated issues of life insurance underwriting and pricing. They must avoid grasping the most politically expedient and seemingly easy solution of prohibiting "genetic discrimination."

References

American Political Network, "Claims Denials: Wall Street Journal Looks at Appeals Options," Am. Health Line 10: 9 (2002).

Andrews, L. B. et al., eds., Assessing Genetic Risks: Implications for Health and Social Policy. Washington, DC: National Academy Press (1994).

Biesecker, B. B., "Privacy in Genetic Counseling," in Genetic Secrets: Protecting Privacy and Confidentiality in the Genetic Era, M. A. Rothstein, ed. New Haven, CT: Yale University Press (1997).

Chabner v. United of Omaha Life Insurance Co., 225 F. 3d 1042 9th Cir. (2000).

Cook, E. D., "Genetics and the British Insurance Industry," J. Med. Ethics 25: 157–162 (1999).

Daniels, N., "The Functions of Insurance and the Fairness of Genetic Underwriting," in Genetics and Life Insurance: Medical Underwriting and Social Policy, M. A. Rothstein, ed. Cambridge: MIT Press (2004).

Dicke, A. A., "The Economics of Risk Selection," in Genetics and Life Insurance: Medical Underwriting and Social Policy, M. A. Rothstein, ed. Cambridge: MIT Press (2004).

Geer, K. P. et al., "Factors Influencing Patients' Decisions to Decline Cancer Genetic Counseling Services," J. Genet. Counsel. 10(1): 25–40 (2001).

Gleeson, R., "Medical Underwriting," in Genetics and Life Insurance: Medical Underwriting and Social Policy, M. A. Rothstein, ed. Cambridge: MIT Press (2004).

Hall, M. A., "Legal Rules and Industry Norms: The Impact of Laws Restricting Health Insurers' Use of Genetic Information," Jurimetrics J. 40: 93–125 (1999).

Hofman, K. J. et al., "Physicians' Knowledge of Genetics and Genetic Tests," Acad. Med. 68: 625–631 (1993).

Holtzman, N. A. and Watson, M. S., eds., "Promoting Safe and Effective Genetic Testing in the United States," final report of the Task Force on Genetic Testing. Baltimore: Johns Hopkins University Press (1998).

Hunter, J. R., "A Consumer Agenda," in Genetics and Life Insurance: Medical Underwriting and Social Policy, M. A. Rothstein, ed. Cambridge: MIT Press (2004).

Investment and Financial Services Association, Ltd. of Australia, Life Insurance and Genetic Testing. Sydney: Investment and Financial Services Association, Ltd. of Australia (2002).

Jerry, R. H., "The Antitrust Implications of Life Insurers' Collaborative Standard Setting," in Genetics and Life Insurance: Medical Underwriting and Social Policy, M. A. Rothstein, ed. Cambridge: MIT Press (2004).

Knoppers, B. M., Godard, B., and Joly, Y., "A Comparative, International Overview," in Genetics and Life Insurance: Medical Underwriting and Social Policy, M. A. Rothstein, ed. Cambridge: MIT Press (2004).

Lemmens, T., "Selective Justice, Genetic Discrimination and Insurance: Should We Single Out Genes in Our Laws?", McGill Law J. 45: 347–375 (2000).

Low, L. et al., "Genetic Discrimination in Life Insurance," Empirical Evidence From a Cross Sectional Survey of Genetic Support Groups in the United Kingdom, Br. Med. J. 317: 1632–1635 (1998).

Lowden, J. A., "Genetic Risks and Mortality Rates," in Genetics and Life Insurance: Medical Underwriting and Social Policy, M. A. Rothstein, ed. Cambridge: MIT Press (2004).

Mariner, W. K., "Independent External Review of Health Maintenance Organizations' Medical Necessity Decisions," N. Engl. J. Med. 347: 2178–2182 (2002).

McEwen, J. E. et al., "A Survey of Medical Directors of Life Insurance Companies Concerning Use of Genetic Information," Am. J. Hum. Genet. 53: 33–45 (1993).

Meyer, R. B., "The Insurer Perspective," in Genetics and Life Insurance: Medical Underwriting and Social Policy, M. A. Rothstein, ed. Cambridge: MIT Press (2004).

Murray, T. H., "Genetic Exceptionalism and 'Future Diaries': Is Genetic Information Different from Other Medical Information?", in Genetic Secrets: Protecting Privacy and Confidentiality in the Genetic Era, M. A. Rothstein ed., New Haven, CT: Yale University Press (1997).

National Conference of State Legislatures, Genetics Policy Report: Insurance Issues. Denver and Washington, D.C.: National Conference of State Legislatures (2001).

National Conference of State Legislatures, Genetics and Life, Disability and Long-term Care Insurance (updated 4/26/02), http://ncsl.org/programs/health/genetics/ndislife.htm (2002).

Ostrager, B. R. and Newman, T. R., Handbook on Insurance Coverage Disputes §12.03[b], [c] Gaithersburg, Md.: Aspen Publishers 10th ed. (2000).

Rothstein, M. A., "Legal Issues in the Medical Assessment of Physical Impairment by Third-party Physicians," J. Legal Med. 5: 503–548 (1984).

Rothstein, M. A., "Genetics, Insurance and the Ethics of Genetic Counseling," Mol. Genet. Med. 3: 159–177 (1993).

Rothstein, M. A., "Genetic Secrets: A Policy Framework," in Genetic Secrets: Protecting Privacy and Confidentiality in the Genetic Era, M. A. Rothstein, ed. New Haven, CT: Yale University Press (1997).

Rothstein, M. A., "Genetic Privacy and Confidentiality: Why They Are so Hard to Protect," J. Law Med. Ethics 26: 198–204 (1998).

Rothstein, M. A., "Why Treating Genetic Information Separately Is a Bad Idea," Tex. Rev. Law Politics 4: 33–37 (1999).

Rothstein, M. A. and Hornung, C. A., "Public Attitudes," in Genetics and Life Insurance: Medical Underwriting and Social Policy, M. A. Rothstein, ed. Cambridge: MIT Press (2004).

Secretary's Advisory Committee on Genetic Testing, Enhancing the Oversight of Genetic Tests: Recommendations of the SACGT, http:www4.od.nih.gov/oba/sacgt.htm (2000).

Social Security Administration, Social Security: Understanding the Benefits, www.ssa.gov/pubs/10024.html/examples (2002).

Subramanian, K. et al., "Estimating Adverse Selection Costs from Genetic Testing for Breast and Ovarian Cancer: The Case of Life Insurance," J. Risk and Insurance 66: 531 (1999).

Uhlmann, W. R. and Terry, S. A., "Perspectives of Consumers and Genetic Professionals," in Genetics and Life Insurance: Medical Underwriting and Social Policy, M. A. Rothstein, ed. Cambridge: MIT Press (2004).

United Kingdom Human Genetics Commission, The Use of Genetic Information in Insurance: Interim Recommendations of the Human Genetics Commission, available at www.hgc.gov.uk/business_publications_statement_01may.htm (2001).

U.S. Chamber of Commerce, The 2001 Employee Benefits Study, Washington, DC: U.S. Chamber of Commerce (2001).

Wachbroit, R., "Genetic Determinism, Genetic Reductionism, and Genetic Essentialism," in Encyclopedia of Ethical, Legal, and Policy Issues in Biotechnology, vol. 1, T. H. Murray and M. J. Mehlman, eds. New York: John Wiley & Sons (2000).

Zick, C. D. et al., "Genetic Testing, Adverse Selection, and the Demand for Life Insurance," Am. J. Med. Genet. 93: 29–39 (2000).

Appendix: Life Insurance and Genetic Testing General Population Survey Questionnaire

Good (morning/afternoon/evening). This is (FIRST & LAST NAME) calling for the University of Louisville School of Medicine. We are conducting a national survey funded by the National Institutes of Health about important health care issues, and your household was randomly selected to represent people living in your area. I would like to invite you to participate.

S1.   First, for this survey, I need to speak with the adult (male/female) member of your household who had the most recent birthday. (Would that be you/Is [he/she] available)?

⟨1⟩ Yes   (CONTINUE)
⟨2⟩ No   (ASK TO SPEAK WITH SELECTED RESPONDENT)
⟨9⟩ RF/DK

Upon Reaching Respondent:

The research we are conducting asks your opinions about different uses of new discoveries in medicine to learn what consumers think about possible uses of genetic information by life insurance companies. The interview takes about 20 minutes, and your participation is completely voluntary. You may decline to participate or end your participation at any time without being subject to any penalty or losing any benefits to which you are otherwise entitled. In addition, you may decline to answer any specific item. All answers you provide will be confidential, meaning that we will not ask you for your name, and a record of the telephone numbers called will not be linked with the responses. In all other respects, confidentiality will be protected to the extent permitted by law. Should any data be published, your identity will not be disclosed.

Although there is the potential for some scientific benefit from this research, you may not derive any personal benefit from your participation. However, your participation in this study poses no risk to you whatsoever. By agreeing to this interview, you acknowledge that the questions you have about the research at this time have been answered in a language you understand. If you have any future questions about this research or your rights as a research subject you can contact the Principal Investigator, Professor Mark Rothstein at (502) 852-4980 or the University of Louisville Human Subjects Committee at (502) 852-5188.

S2.   Would you be willing to participate in this important study?

⟨1⟩ Yes   (CONTINUE)
⟨2⟩ No   (THANK & TERMINATE)

First, would you say your health is ... (READ LIST)

⟨1⟩ Excellent
⟨2⟩ Very Good
⟨3⟩ Good
⟨4⟩ Fair, or
⟨5⟩ Poor?
⟨7⟩ Refused
⟨8⟩ Unsure

Some differences among people are passed down from parents to their children through genes. Some genes determine things like hair color and height. Other genes can even be used to predict who will get sick and how long a person might live.

Do you believe that life insurance companies should have access to the genetic information of people who are applying for policies?

⟨1⟩ Yes
⟨2⟩ No
⟨7⟩ Refused
⟨8⟩ Unsure

Genetic testing is a quick and painless procedure, such as having a blood test or simply brushing the inside of your mouth with a cotton swab.

Genetic tests are done for different reasons and give different kinds of information. For the rest of this interview, we are going to be talking about genetic tests that are done for two reasons: First, genetic tests that are done to help doctors determine if you **currently** have a serious disease; and second, genetic tests that are done to determine if you are at risk of getting a serious disease **in the future**. I would like to find out how likely you would be to have a genetic test for each of the two reasons.

A. First, how likely would you be to have a genetic test to help determine if you **currently** have a serious disease? Would you be ... (READ CATEGORIES)

⟨1⟩ Very Likely
⟨2⟩ Somewhat Likely
⟨3⟩ Somewhat Unlikely
⟨4⟩ Very Unlikely
⟨7⟩ Refused
⟨8⟩ Unsure

B. And, how likely would you be to have a genetic test to help determine if you are at risk of getting a serious disease **in the future**? Would you be ... (READ CATEGORIES)

⟨1⟩ Very Likely
⟨2⟩ Somewhat Likely
⟨3⟩ Somewhat Unlikely
⟨4⟩ Very Unlikely
⟨7⟩ Refused
⟨8⟩ Unsure

Now I would like to ask some questions specifically about life insurance. First, do you currently have any life insurance through your employer, through a professional association, union or other organization, through military service or that you purchased directly on your own?

⟨1⟩ Yes   (ASK A)
⟨2⟩ No   (SKIP TO Q6)
⟨7⟩ Refused   (SKIP TO Q6)
⟨8⟩ Unsure   (SKIP TO Q6)

IF YES, ASK A1–A5. ELSE SKIP TO Q6:

Through which of the following sources do you have life insurance?

	Yes	No	RF	DK
A1. Through your job or your spouse's job?	1	2	7	8
A2. Through a professional association or union?	1	2	7	8
A3. Through military service?	1	2	7	8
A4. That you purchased on your own?	1	2	7	8
A5. Through any other organization or source?	1	2	7	8

Specify: —————

People have life insurance for a number of different reasons. I'm going to read a list of three reasons people have life insurance and ask you to tell me which one is the main reason **you** have life insurance. The **main reason** I have life insurance is ...

⟨1⟩ To pay for my burial and other final expenses
⟨2⟩ To give my family and me peace of mind that they will have some money if I die
⟨3⟩ Or, to leave money to my family when I die
⟨4⟩ None of the above (VOLUNTEERED)
⟨7⟩ Refused
⟨8⟩ Unsure

Now I am going to read some statements about insurance and ask you to tell me whether you strongly agree, agree, have no opinion, disagree or strongly disagree with each one. The first statement is ... [BLOCK ROTATE A & B WITH C & D]

A.   Everyone needs **health** insurance. Do you ...

⟨1⟩ Strongly Agree
⟨2⟩ Agree
⟨3⟩ Have No Opinion
⟨4⟩ Disagree
⟨5⟩ Strongly Disagree
⟨7⟩ Refused
⟨8⟩ Unsure

B. Everyone has a right to **health** insurance. Do you ...

⟨1⟩ Strongly Agree
⟨2⟩ Agree
⟨3⟩ Have No Opinion
⟨4⟩ Disagree
⟨5⟩ Strongly Disagree
⟨7⟩ Refused
⟨8⟩ Unsure

C. Everyone needs **life** insurance. Do you ...

⟨1⟩ Strongly Agree
⟨2⟩ Agree
⟨3⟩ Have No Opinion
⟨4⟩ Disagree
⟨5⟩ Strongly Disagree
⟨7⟩ Refused
⟨8⟩ Unsure

D. Everyone has a right to **life** insurance. Do you ...

⟨1⟩ Strongly Agree
⟨2⟩ Agree
⟨3⟩ Have No Opinion
⟨4⟩ Disagree
⟨5⟩ Strongly Disagree
⟨7⟩ Refused
⟨8⟩ Unsure

Have you ever applied for life insurance or tried to increase your life insurance coverage and been rejected?

⟨1⟩ Yes
⟨2⟩ No
⟨7⟩ Refused
⟨8⟩ Unsure

Does anyone else in your household have life insurance?

⟨1⟩ Yes
⟨2⟩ No

⟨7⟩ Refused
⟨8⟩ Unsure

ASK EVERYONE:

9. As you may know, life insurance companies use a range of information including your age, personal health history, risk factors such as smoking or drinking, and other health information to decide whether to offer you life insurance and, if so, to set the price you pay. I am going to read two statements about the methods life insurance companies use to set prices and ask you to tell me whether you strongly agree, agree, have no opinion, disagree or strongly disagree with each one. The first is ...

ROTATE:

A.   Everyone who is the same age should be able to get life insurance for the same price regardless of their health. Do you ...

⟨1⟩ Strongly Agree
⟨2⟩ Agree
⟨3⟩ Have No Opinion
⟨4⟩ Disagree
⟨5⟩ Strongly Disagree
⟨7⟩ Refused
⟨8⟩ Unsure

B.   To make prices fair for everyone, life insurance companies should take a person's current health and risk factors like smoking or drinking into account when they are setting prices for their life insurance. Do you ...

⟨1⟩ Strongly Agree
⟨2⟩ Agree
⟨3⟩ Have No Opinion
⟨4⟩ Disagree
⟨5⟩ Strongly Disagree
⟨7⟩ Refused
⟨8⟩ Unsure

Now I would like to find out what you think life insurance companies might do if they have access to genetic information. If a life insurance company has access to the genetic information of someone applying for a life insurance policy, do you think they would be likely to ...

	Yes	No	RF	DK
A. Refuse to sell the policy	1	2	7	8
B. Agree to sell the policy at the regular price	1	2	7	8
C. Agree to sell the policy at a higher price	1	2	7	8
D. Agree to sell the policy at a lower price	1	2	7	8

Now I am going to read two statements about what **consumers** might do if they have access to genetic information and life insurance companies don't. Please tell me if you strongly agree, agree, have no opinion, disagree or strongly disagree with each one. The first is ...

A.   If they got a genetic test result saying that they were more likely to get a serious illness, many people would withhold the test results from a life insurance company. Do you ...

⟨1⟩ Strongly Agree
⟨2⟩ Agree
⟨3⟩ Have No Opinion
⟨4⟩ Disagree
⟨5⟩ Strongly Disagree
⟨7⟩ Refused
⟨8⟩ Unsure

[PROGRAMMER: SET TO RANDOMLY SELECT B1 **OR** B2]

B1.   It would be wrong to withhold genetic information from a life insurance company. Do you ...

⟨1⟩ Strongly Agree
⟨2⟩ Agree
⟨3⟩ Have No Opinion
⟨4⟩ Disagree

⟨5⟩ Strongly Disagree
⟨7⟩ Refused
⟨8⟩ Unsure

B2.   It would **not** be wrong to withhold genetic information from a life insurance company. Do you ...

⟨1⟩ Strongly Agree
⟨2⟩ Agree
⟨3⟩ Have No Opinion
⟨4⟩ Disagree
⟨5⟩ Strongly Disagree
⟨7⟩ Refused
⟨8⟩ Unsure

C.   I am concerned that people who get unfavorable genetic test results would buy large life insurance policies and drive up the costs for everybody. Do you ...

⟨1⟩ Strongly Agree
⟨2⟩ Agree
⟨3⟩ Have No Opinion
⟨4⟩ Disagree
⟨5⟩ Strongly Disagree
⟨7⟩ Refused
⟨8⟩ Unsure

12. If a medical test indicated that you, personally, had an increased chance of getting cancer or heart disease in the next 10 years, would you be likely or unlikely to (buy/buy more) (ITEM)?

ROTATE:

A.   Health insurance?

⟨1⟩ Likely
⟨2⟩ Unlikely
⟨7⟩ Refused
⟨8⟩ Unsure

B. Life insurance?

⟨1⟩ Likely
⟨2⟩ Unlikely
⟨7⟩ Refused
⟨8⟩ Unsure

C. Long term care or nursing home insurance?

⟨1⟩ Likely
⟨2⟩ Unlikely
⟨7⟩ Refused
⟨8⟩ Unsure

D. Disability insurance that would pay a portion of your wages if you could not work due to accident or illness?

⟨1⟩ Likely
⟨2⟩ Unlikely
⟨7⟩ Refused
⟨8⟩ Unsure

Are you concerned that, as scientists learn more about genetics, there is likely to be genetic discrimination?

⟨1⟩ Yes   (ASK A)
⟨2⟩ No   (SKIP TO Q14)
⟨7⟩ Refused   (SKIP TO Q14)
⟨8⟩ Unsure   (SKIP TO Q14)

IF YES ASK:

A. I am going to ask you to compare your concern about genetic discrimination with your concerns about other issues. Would you say you are more concerned, less concerned or equally concerned about genetic discrimination as you are about ...

	More	Equal	Less	RF	DK
ROTATE:					
A1. Cloning?	1	2	3	7	8
A2. Crime?	1	2	3	7	8

A3. The Economy?	1	2	3	7	8
A4. The Environment?	1	2	3	7	8
A5. Access to Health Care?	1	2	3	7	8
A6. Taxes?	1	2	3	7	8
A7. Terrorism?	1	2	3	7	8

ASK EVERYONE:

14. How much trust would you have in each of the following groups to keep genetic information private? First,...

ROTATE:

A.   How much trust would you have in the federal government to keep genetic information private? Would you have ...

⟨1⟩ A Great Deal of Trust
⟨2⟩ Some Trust
⟨3⟩ Some Lack of Trust
⟨4⟩ No Trust
⟨7⟩ Refused
⟨8⟩ Unsure

B.   How much trust would you have in drug companies to keep genetic information private? Would you have ...

⟨1⟩ A Great Deal of Trust
⟨2⟩ Some Trust
⟨3⟩ Some Lack of Trust
⟨4⟩ No Trust
⟨7⟩ Refused
⟨8⟩ Unsure

C.   How much trust would you have in universities and medical schools to keep genetic information private? Would you have ...

⟨1⟩ A Great Deal of Trust
⟨2⟩ Some Trust

⟨3⟩ Some Lack of Trust
⟨4⟩ No Trust
⟨7⟩ Refused
⟨8⟩ Unsure

D.   How much trust would you have in organizations like the American Cancer Society and the March of Dimes to keep genetic information private? Would you have ...

⟨1⟩ A Great Deal of Trust
⟨2⟩ Some Trust
⟨3⟩ Some Lack of Trust
⟨4⟩ No Trust
⟨7⟩ Refused
⟨8⟩ Unsure

E.   How much trust would you have in health insurance companies to keep genetic information private? Would you have ...

⟨1⟩ A Great Deal of Trust
⟨2⟩ Some Trust
⟨3⟩ Some Lack of Trust
⟨4⟩ No Trust
⟨7⟩ Refused
⟨8⟩ Unsure

F.   How much trust would you have in life insurance companies to keep genetic information private? Would you have ...

⟨1⟩ A Great Deal of Trust
⟨2⟩ Some Trust
⟨3⟩ Some Lack of Trust
⟨4⟩ No Trust
⟨7⟩ Refused
⟨8⟩ Unsure

15. Now I am going to read some general statements about life insurance and genetic testing and ask you to tell me whether you agree, disagree or have no opinion. The first is ...

ROTATE:

A.   Life insurance companies should be allowed to require all applicants to take a genetic test.

⟨1⟩ Agree
⟨2⟩ No Opinion
⟨3⟩ Disagree
⟨7⟩ Refused
⟨8⟩ Unsure

B.   Life insurance companies should not be allowed to use either the results of genetic tests or other genetic information.

⟨1⟩ Agree
⟨2⟩ No Opinion
⟨3⟩ Disagree
⟨7⟩ Refused
⟨8⟩ Unsure

C.   Life insurance companies should be able to use genetic information from existing medical records, but they should not be allowed to require applicants to take a genetic test.

⟨1⟩ Agree
⟨2⟩ No Opinion
⟨3⟩ Disagree
⟨7⟩ Refused
⟨8⟩ Unsure

Do you believe that life insurance companies should have access to the genetic information of people who are applying for policies?

⟨1⟩ Yes
⟨2⟩ No
⟨7⟩ Refused
⟨8⟩ Unsure

D1.   Now for some background questions, and we will be finished. First, including yourself, how many people live in your household full time?

NUMBER: ____ ____

⟨97⟩ Refused
⟨98⟩ Unsure

IF MORE THAN ONE, ASK:

D2.   How many of these are age 18 and older?
NUMBER: ____ ____

⟨97⟩ Refused
⟨98⟩ Unsure

D3.   What is your age?
AGE: ____ ____

⟨97⟩ Refused
⟨98⟩ Unsure

D4.   What is the highest grade of school or college you completed?
(DO NOT READ LIST)

⟨01⟩ 8ᵗʰ Grade or Less	100	4.8
⟨02⟩ Some High School	148	7.1
⟨03⟩ High School Graduate	652	31.2
⟨04⟩ Trade or Technical School	57	2.7
⟨05⟩ Some College	569	27.2
⟨06⟩ Bachelor's Degree	367	17.5
⟨07⟩ Graduate Degree	184	8.8
⟨97⟩ Refused	8	0.4
⟨98⟩ Unsure	7	0.3

D5.   Are you currently ...   (READ LIST)

⟨1⟩ Married	1149	54.9
⟨2⟩ Widowed	206	9.8
⟨3⟩ Separated or Divorced	253	12.1
⟨4⟩ In a Domestic Partnership, or	87	4.1
⟨5⟩ Single/Never Married?	387	18.5
⟨7⟩ Refused	11	0.5
⟨8⟩ Unsure	1	0.0

D6.   Are you currently ...   (READ LIST)

⟨01⟩ Employed Full Time	1045	49.9
⟨02⟩ Employed Part Time	182	8.7
⟨03⟩ Unemployed	171	8.2
⟨04⟩ Retired	403	19.3
⟨05⟩ Disabled	93	4.4
⟨06⟩ A Student, or	74	3.5
⟨06⟩ Something else? *(Specify)*	119	5.7

⟨07⟩ Refused	6	0.3
⟨08⟩ Unsure	1	0.0

D7.   Do you live in ...   (READ LIST)

⟨1⟩ A large city with a population over 100,000	713	34.0
⟨2⟩ A suburban area outside a large city	370	17.7
⟨3⟩ A small city with a population of less than 100,000	538	25.7
⟨4⟩ A rural or farm area?	443	21.2
⟨7⟩ Refused	7	0.3
⟨8⟩ Unsure	23	1.1

D8.   Do you consider yourself ...

⟨1⟩ Caucasian or White, Non-Hispanic	1488	71.1
⟨2⟩ Black or African-American	261	12.5
⟨3⟩ Hispanic	268	12.8
⟨4⟩ Asian or Asian-American, or	76	3.6
⟨5⟩ Something else? *(Specify)*		

⟨7⟩ Refused

⟨8⟩ Unsure

D9.   What language do you speak most often at home?   (DO NOT READ LIST)

⟨01⟩ English	1842	88.0
⟨02⟩ Spanish	179	8.5
⟨03⟩ Chinese (Mandarin or Cantonese)	48	2.3
⟨04⟩ Vietnamese	5	0.3
⟨05⟩ Korean	1	0.0
⟨06⟩ Other Asian Language *(Specify)*	4	0.2

―――――――――――

⟨07⟩ Other Language (Non-Asian) *(Specify)*	14	0.7

―――――――

⟨97⟩ Refused		
⟨98⟩ Unsure	1	0.1

D10.   In what country were you born?   (DO NOT READ LIST)

⟨01⟩ United States (including Alaska and Hawaii)	1794	85.7
⟨02⟩ U.S. Territory (Puerto Rico, Guam, etc.)	9	0.4
⟨02⟩ Mexico	119	5.7
⟨03⟩ Cuba	7	0.3
⟨04⟩ China	35	1.7
⟨05⟩ Taiwan	7	0.3
⟨06⟩ Vietnam	8	0.4
⟨07⟩ Korea	1	0.1
⟨08⟩ Other *(Specify)*	107	5.1

―――――――

⟨97⟩ Refused	4	0.2
⟨98⟩ Unsure	2	0.1

D11.   What is your religious preference, if any? Is it ...   (READ LIST)

⟨01⟩ Protestant	789	37.7
⟨02⟩ Catholic	528	25.2
⟨03⟩ Jewish	23	1.1
⟨04⟩ Mormon	26	1.3
⟨05⟩ Islam	11	0.5

⟨06⟩ Buddhist   21   1.0
⟨07⟩ Other Religion   *(Specify)*   366   17.5

_____

⟨08⟩ No Religious Preference?   300   14.3
⟨97⟩ Refused   26   1.2
⟨98⟩ Unsure   3   0.1

D12. Was your 2000 total household income; that is, income for all members of your household during 2000 ... (READ LIST)

⟨1⟩ Under $25,000   463   22.1
⟨2⟩ $25,000 to $49,999   564   26.9
⟨3⟩ $50,000 to $74,999   391   18.7
⟨4⟩ $75,000 to $99,999, or   180   8.6
⟨5⟩ $100,000 or more?   200   9.5
⟨7⟩ Refused   187   9.0
⟨8⟩ Unsure   108   5.1

D13. These last two questions are about your personal health history and you can feel free not to answer them. First, have you ever had a genetic test?

⟨1⟩ Yes   165   7.9
⟨2⟩ No   1869   89.3
⟨7⟩ Refused   22   1.1
⟨8⟩ Unsure   38   1.8

D14. Has a doctor ever told you that you are at increased risk of getting a serious disease like heart disease or cancer in the future?

⟨1⟩ Yes   329   15.7
⟨2⟩ No.   1734   82.9
⟨7⟩ Refused   23   1.1
⟨8⟩ Unsure   6   0.3

That concludes our interview. Thank you for your time and help with this important research effort.

D15.   Interviewer Record:

⟨1⟩ Male	981	46.9
⟨2⟩ Female	1112	53.1

D16.   Language of Interview:

⟨1⟩ English	1914	91.4
⟨2⟩ Spanish	137	6.5
⟨3⟩ Chinese	39	1.9
⟨4⟩ Vietnamese	4	0.2

Index

Prognostic genetic tests, 39–40
Prohibitive approach to genetic
  testing, 184–185, 255–256
Protective value of genetic tests,
  98–100
Public opinion
  about genetic discrimination relative
    to other issues, 20–22
  on expected actions of life insurance
    companies, 7–11
  on genetics and insurance under-
    writing, 1–2, 148–150, 234–235
  on insurance as a right, 148,
    217–219
  on insurance purchasing behavior
    and genetic information, 11–16
  and interest in purchasing all forms
    of insurance, 14–15
  on the need for life insurance, 22–24
  on possible regulation of life
    insurers' use of genetic informa-
    tion, 16–20
  prior research of, 2–5
  on sharing of genetic information,
    2–3

Rasmusen, Eric, 55–56
Rates
  affordable, 239–240
  flat extras in, 82
  preferred class, 64–66, 257–258,
    258–259
  standard and substandard, 54–55
  and time value of money, 59
  using insured mortality tables,
    81–82, 228
  using results of genetic tests to
    obtain coverage at regular,
    258–259
Red-lining, 129
Requirements, medical underwriting,
  87–88
Research
  documenting genetic discrimination,
    151–156
  on expected action of life insurance
    companies, 7–11

focus groups, 5
public opinion on sharing of genetic
  information, 2–5
telephone interview, 5–7, 155
Restrictions on the use of genetic
  information in different countries,
  178–181t, 221–223
Risk classification, 233. *See also*
  Underwriting, medical
  adverse selection and, 29–31
  concentration, 63
  economic analysis in, 49–51
  fairness in, 31–32, 40–41, 240
  impact of medical advances on,
    88–89
  importance of, 33–34
  and mortality, 82–83
  myths related to genetics and, 40
  operation of economic incentives
    and, 32–33
  protection of financial soundness by,
    29
  in regulated and competitive envi-
    ronments, 75–76
  regulation, 75–76
  unobserved relative risk and, 64–
    66
  use of genetic information in, 34–36,
    95–98, 141–143
Rothstein, Mark A., 147
Rule of reason, 198–199, 200

*Sandy River Nursing Care v. Aetna
  Casualty*, 203
Secondary markets for life insurance,
  61–62
*Securities and Exchange Commission
  v. National Securities, Inc.*,
  206–207
Self-regulation, insurance industry,
  203–204
Senior settlements, 61–62
Shadow charts, 161–162
Sherman Act, 196–198, 213
Signaling in applications, 60
Single nucleotide polymorphisms
  (SNPs), 102, 105